it's not about cancer
it's about you

Conquer Your Dreams
is
Crying Your Gift
of Life!

it's not about cancer
it's about you

six reasons to
keep living and enjoying
your gift of life

Larry S. Cockerel

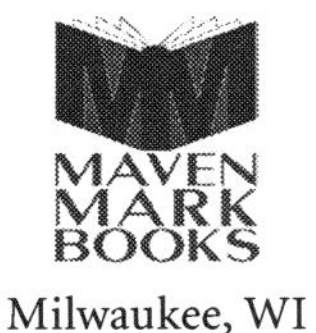

MAVEN
MARK
BOOKS

Milwaukee, WI

Published by
MavenMark Books
A division of HenschelHAUS Publishing, Inc.
2625 S. Greeley St. Suite 201
Milwaukee, WI 53207
www.HenschelHAUSbooks.com

Please contact the author or the publisher regarding quantity discounts.

Also available in Kindle and other e-book formats.

ISBN: 978-159598-120-2

Publisher's Cataloging-In-Publication Data
(Prepared by The Donohue Group, Inc.)

Cockerel, Larry S.
    It's not about cancer, it's about you : six reasons to keep living
and enjoying your gift of life / Larry S. Cockerel.

     p. : ill. ; cm.

    Issued also as an ebook.
    ISBN: 978-1-59598-120-2 (pbk)
    ISBN: 978-1-59598-119-6 (hardcover)

    1. Cockerel, Larry S.--Health. 2. Cancer--Patients--Conduct of
life. 3. Cancer--Psychological aspects. I. Title. II. Title: It's
about you

RC265.6.C62 C62 2011
362.19/6994/0092   2011931430

Cover and interior design by Andrew Welyczko.

Printed in the United States of America.

This book is dedicated to all the courageous men, women,
and children who have been diagnosed with cancer,
or who have a loved one who has been diagnosed with
this unwanted life experience.

My hope is that you live your dreams, love your life,
and enjoy your gift of life each day.

I honor and salute you!

◆　◆　◆

contents

foreword

You are most likely reading this book because you or a loved one is at a crossroads in life. You are looking for answers. You are looking for courage. You have started on a journey you hoped you would never have to make. But now you do.

This journey is unlike any other. It's a journey of personal change. It's a journey of personal discovery. No two journeys are ever the same.

My friend and colleague, Larry Cockerel, has made this journey.

This book is his story.

Larry is one of the most optimistic and enthusiastic people I know. When confronted with a setback or challenge, he argues for possibilities, not limitations. When he speaks to audiences, trains organizations, or coaches individuals, he does exactly the same thing: he argues for possibilities, not limitations.

I've known Larry for over ten years as a professional speaker. We have appeared together at a number of conferences throughout Wisconsin and the Midwest. We really got to know each other during the time when we served together on the Board of Directors for the National Speakers Association of Wisconsin. I had just concluded my term as President and Larry had just become President. The year was 2008.

2008 was a year of painful change. The markets crashed. The global financial crisis took center stage. Lives were turned upside-down. The fallout from these catastrophic events continues to this day.

When a crisis strikes, sometimes it can appear there is no way out. It can seem like there are no choices or options. When the sky is gray and storm clouds on the horizon are heading in your direction, they will often pass without incident. Why? Because most of the things we worry about never happen.

But what happens when those storm clouds turn into life-changing or potentially life-threatening events? Those are the moments in life that require us to sit up, take notice and pursue an altogether different course of action than we might have otherwise considered. Those are the transformational moments in life when change really happens.

Lots of people fear change, resist change, or attempt to avoid change. Many people think that if change is good, then someone else should try it first.

I believe change is neither good nor bad; it simply is. You make it one or the other by your choices and actions.

Breakthroughs can happen at any time.

Even now.

Robert Ian, CEO
Change Management International LLC
www.conquerchange.com

preface

The timing could not have been any better. Fall in the Rockies. It was the week of October 12, 2007, the week that Debbie and I always do our best to take a vacation, a sort of anniversary get-away. This time, the Rockies were our destination. We had it all planned out: we'd reserved a nice bed-and-breakfast at Blue Skies Inn B&B in Manitou Springs, CO at the base of Pikes Peak, the Harley had been reserved to rent, and we'd looked at hiking and other activities to fill those precious seven days.

The first attraction on the "vacation bucket list" was the summit of Pikes Peak, more than 14,000 feet up the winding road under those awesome blue Colorado skies. We took the clog train ride to the top of Pikes Peak, which was a lifetime experience we both enjoyed. From the start, Debbie and I knew this was going to be one of our favorite vacations. The weather was perfect: blue skies, mid-seventies, light breeze, and barely even a cloud in sight.

Debbie and I hiked along a number of the state park's trails and smaller mountains. Getting out in the fresh air was wonderful. We did the Harley thing for a whole day, heading west into the mountains on a beautiful, powerful, black Harley Road King. I've been a Harley guy forever, and fortunately, Debbie loves the riding as much as I do. We followed the

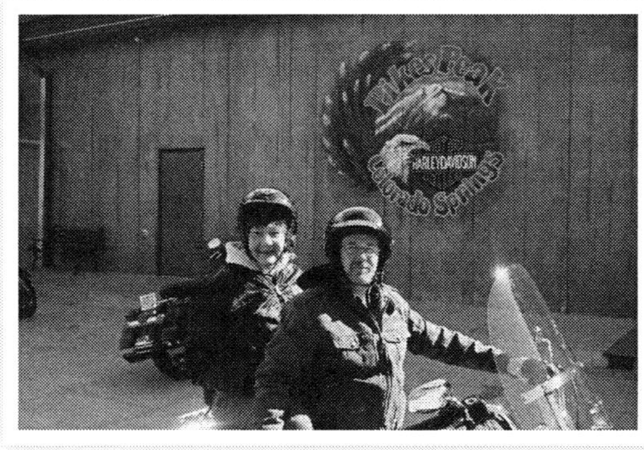

winding road along the Arkansas River as we headed back to Colorado Springs. The small towns we passed reminded us of a good ole cowboy movie, with the mountains peacefully surrounding the towns. We just wanted to keep riding, truly were enjoying the trip.

We had a packed vacation planned and midway through, headed to Rocky Mountain National Park. Folks, let me tell you, if you haven't visited that beautiful place, put it on the calendar. The park turned out to be the best part of the vacation; the ride out and then the drive up the highest paved highway in North America (Trail Ridge Road) was the best. The curves were scary; the views were spectacular. Debbie and I both felt this was a life-changing experience of true freedom and the magnificence of this amazing planet.

Another reason the trip was a life-changing experience was because something was growing in me without my being aware of it. This vacation had it all: great sites, lots of activity, wonderful food! It also had something I really didn't know much about at the time: a small lump on the right side of my neck. I had first noticed the small bump or lump just before we left Milwaukee. I was a little curious about the lump, but the guy who never got sick, never had a stitch or broken bone, thought it couldn't be that serious. Maybe it was even an allergic reaction to something I'd eaten. I never gave a thought to cancer or anything to that degree. Who knew? The truth was it didn't slow us down.

After we returned to Milwaukee, still floating on the terrific and relaxing week, however, that little lump continued to grow. It started to become noticeable. There wasn't really any pain, but I knew something wasn't quite right.

The year 2008 started the process of discovery. By mid-year, I knew I needed to see a doctor, and guess what? I didn't have one. I never believed in looking for trouble and had never needed a doctor until that point. By July 2008, it seemed that the lump was alive, that it had a personality, and it kept getting larger. My gut feeling wasn't good. I was doing my best to stay as positive and optimistic as usual. The goal became finding a physician and trying to determine what the thing was, good or bad. After some searching, Debbie and I found one. The tests, scans, and blood tests began. Then we moved into the biopsy phase to figure out if the lump was benign or not. The whole deal was getting a little worrisome for "Mr. Enthusiasm" at that point, but I knew I had to keep moving forward.

The scary-sounding "needle biopsy" was scheduled. Debbie arranged her time to be with me and we were off to experience something I had never, ever done in my life. Initially, the doctor said it would be about three sticks, or maybe five. Then the number of sticks became six. I got a little dizzy from all that sticking. The whole ordeal was not my thing: the needles, the blood, the pressure, and stress of the unknown.

One ever-so-long week later, I received a call from the doctor saying that it was all okay and there was nothing to worry about. We just needed to get it out, even though it appeared to be benign. My first thought: "WOW! I'm good to go. No cancer. I'm better." I felt better just getting that call.

I set up an appointment with the clinic's head and neck specialist, an otolaryngologist, or ENT (ear, nose, throat) doctor, to hear his pitch on what needed to be done. Believe me, I was all ears. "Cut the lump out, come back in ten days, and get the stitches out, no worries." All the while, my gut was saying, "Something isn't right with all this small talk." It all sounded a little too easy to me.

I shared my uneasiness with Debbie while describing what the first physician had told me about the surgery. I went back about two weeks later to meet with the "specialist" to review the process with a clearer mind. However, just two days before going into that meeting, I received a letter from my insurance company informing me that the specialist and the clinic I had been going to were being dropped on December 30, 2008, about six months away. Was this fate or luck?

As the salesman that I am, I went into my sales mode to question the diagnosis, ready to test the motive of the physician. I went back to the doc and the clinic with all my guns loaded. Maybe it was my intuition, or maybe God was speaking to me. Whatever it was, I knew deep down something wasn't right. The physician started explaining the procedure to me again. To me, it still sounded way too simple. I told him about the letter I'd gotten. Without even blinking an eye, he turned away from his computer and looked me straight in the eye, saying that then we needed to hurry up and get this scheduled and completed before the end of year.

My immediate thought was, "You're fired!" So I took action and made the decision. There was no more time to be wasted. I needed to get a second opinion and seek out another head and neck doctor.

I went home really confused and told Debbie I didn't know what to do. One thing I was sure about, though: that "doctor" wasn't going to put a scalpel to any part of my body.

The lump kept growing, so I knew I had to do something. I could feel that something wasn't right. My energy was way down, I had lost a lot of weight, and by fall of 2008, the lump had grown to the size of a small orange.

Nevertheless, I kept pushing my business, making appointments, and giving talks. I had a meeting scheduled with the president of our National Speakers Association of Wisconsin Chapter, Robert Ian, who is also a good friend and mentor. I was truly looking forward to catching up with Robert and finding out what was going on in the chapter. I had been involved in the Wisconsin chapter for nine years and was getting ready to step up to the president's role to support the growth of the chapter. I was ready to give back. I'd always been a giver, doing my best to help others from my experiences just as I am doing now with my cancer experience.

Robert and I met at Taco John's in Madison. It turned out to be much more than a lunch and a casual meeting of the minds. Robert asked me about the lump and I shared what had happened in Milwaukee. Robert told me that his wife had spent the last fourteen years working with one of the best head and neck surgeons in the United States, right there at the University of Wisconsin–Madison. On the spot, Robert called his wife and got me the number and the name of the surgeon. I was on my way!

You know how you feel when you're not in control and something much bigger than you is in the driver's seat? Well, having the lump on my neck was one of those times. That day with Robert, I believe God was in control. God's plan was in action and Robert was the messenger. What was supposed to be a business meeting turned out to be the meeting of my life. My new journey had begun.

I drove home as quickly as I could. Debbie and I started the process of learning as much as we could about neck cancer, the proposed surgeon and UW Hospital. We did our research and this was the place, noted as one of the best in the country with respect to head and neck cancer and treatments.

A few days later, I had an appointment. What a difference between UW Hospital in Madison and the clinic where I had gotten all the original scans and tests. When I rolled into the parking deck of UW Hospital and walked through those big revolving doors, I knew it was for real. With all my heart, I wished Debbie could have been at my side, but also I knew that I needed to do this on my own. I was ready for the journey. My number had been picked and my time to step up and get this done was now.

Over the months that had passed between my first noticing the lump in October, the initial diagnosis, and these visits with the UW doctor, the small lump in my neck had grown much larger—it was like a large grapefruit sticking out of the side of my neck. Two meetings later, another uncomfortable needle biopsy, and "BAM," it all came together. On December 11, 2008, the head and neck surgeon told me that after the biopsy, the radiology team would review the results and that he would call me. At that moment I knew. I could feel it. I could see it in his face. It was cancer.

I got on the highway heading toward Milwaukee and not more than forty minutes after I pulled out of the hospital parking lot, my cell phone rang. Yes, it was "the call."

We all get "the call" at some time in our lives, the call that can completely and utterly change our lives. The call that will take us down a new path, redirect our journey, our plans. I answered. It was the surgeon telling me the lump was indeed cancer, which he called "squamous cell carcinoma." Apparently that kind of cancer is about 90 percent of all head and neck cancers, and 700,000 are diagnosed every year.

The doctor went on to explain that it was a Stage 4 tumor, unknown source. He then recommended that we should schedule surgery as soon as possible. The conversation didn't last more than ten minutes. I never took my eyes off the road, just listened, asked a few questions, and kept moving forward to my destination—home.

My mind kept repeating: "I have cancer—a stage-4-type cancer—and I need to have surgery ASAP." My heart knew. It didn't feel like a surprise to me; I just knew. I did not pull over and think "Oh, my God, I'm dying." Nor did I pull over to cry my eyes out with pity. Nope, I just kept driving, my eyes on the highway, moving forward with the right attitude. My first thoughts were, "I'm not giving in or giving up. What am I going to do with this cancer? How can I turn this experience into something good?"

Gripping the steering wheel of my 2005 red Dodge Magnum, right then and there, I made the decision that I was not going to let this cancer thing control my life. I just kept driving, heading home. I was keeping to my course. That day did begin to change my life. I had a new journey ahead of me, a new chapter in my life. That day opened my eyes; it got me excited, scared and ready.

For the next two hours, I put together an inspirational speech about recovery in my head. I thought about how I could encourage others. I was already thinking of the positive outcomes, rather than the negatives that cancer can bring. It's not my nature to think in a negative or pessimistic way. I never have been anything other than an optimist. I wasn't going to start being pessimistic when I needed to be on my best game.

This book also had its beginning during those 100 miles between Madison and Cedarburg. I was actually getting excited about writing a book, something that could help others. I tried to come up with a title. The first one that popped into my head was "The Journey." "The Journey" seemed a little too normal a title, but it sounded good to me. It would be about my journey of recovery and hope.

My thoughts were all over the road that day, but better than me all over the road! I needed to stop at Wal-Mart and get a few home supplies—cat litter, paper towels, and other things. My usual modus operandi is: "Get in, get my stuff, and get home." But something bigger than me happened while at

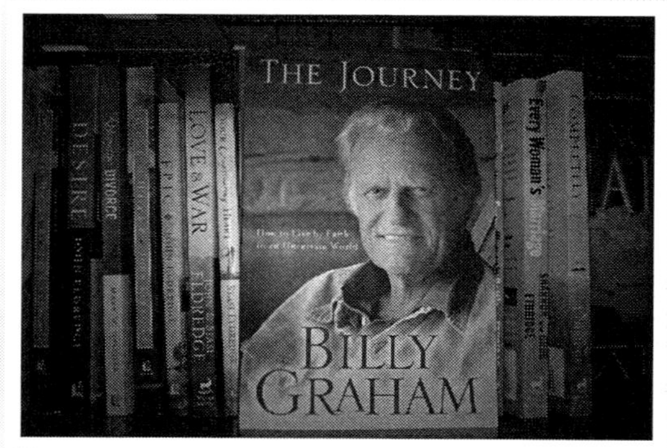

Wal-Mart. I ended up in the book aisle with no intention of looking at or buying any book. Suddenly, I found myself parked right in front of a title, *The Journey*, by Billy Graham. Those very words had been rumbling around in my head for the past two hours and 100 miles. In a flash, I knew that this book was meant for me to read, not write. God was leading my thoughts and paving the road for me to travel, my journey!

You'd better believe I bought the book. I'm not sure I really had an option. God was in control and I knew it. My journey truly began that day. As I left that Wal-Mart, I felt no fear. Instead, I knew deep down that it was time to get excited about getting this cancer out of me as soon as I could. What a day! What was next?

Initially, I thought Debbie and I would have time to make decisions, to ask questions, search the Internet, and find answers. We did research online, in books, wherever. We were just trying to understand why, where it had come from, how it had gotten into my neck? Debbie put in hours of Google research about the operation, radiation, the feeding tube process, and on and on. More information than I really wanted. I just wanted to get the surgery over with and begin the therapy process. There were so many questions; there didn't seem to be an end in sight.

I knew the growth was getting bigger; it was alive and growing inside me, wanting to take over my life and control it. After meeting with the experts, the surgery date was set for January 27, 2009, and radiation treatments would start four weeks after.

❖　❖　❖

What Appears To Be BIG Gets Even BIGGER When You Focus On It!

When I say big, I mean big! The word cancer looks scary. When you say the word, it sounds scary. It's a big thing, a big disappointment, a big ugly label. "I have cancer." There is nothing little about this disease. It's a heavy load to carry, the big white elephant on your shoulders. It's a burden no one wishes for themselves or anyone else.

I found that it's complicated, too. There was and still is a lot of stuff to learn and understand. Like big complicated words, phrases, and big decisions to make. This thing was bigger than Debbie and me. We have truly been challenged: our relationship, our lifestyle, and our faith. It was time to step up to the plate and face my giant.

January 2009 came fast and Debbie and I had appointments to meet the surgeon and his team to discuss the operation. The first team meeting on January 6, 2009, was one of the scariest and most overwhelming gatherings that Debbie and I had ever experienced. Packed into a small hospital meeting room were seven people, all with a mission and a purpose: Debbie and me, members of the oncology team, radiation doctors, and the "feeding tube people."

Debbie's fears were tangible. She was worried about losing our home, my losing my job, losing me—normal thoughts under the circumstances. Me? I was thinking about losing my hair!

I also realized something bigger was in that room with us: God's presence.

After what seemed an eternity, the forty-five minute meeting ended and Debbie and I went through a battery of other appointments to discuss treatments after surgery. Those people didn't slow down! The treatments recommended were: radiation treatments (30), every day for six weeks, 5 days a week, as well as weekly chemotherapy treatments. WOW! That was a lot to take in for a guy who had never been sick, was rarely in pain, and had never had a broken bone or even stitches throughout his 50 years.

Christmas was upon us, so off to Cabot, Arkansas to spend Christmas with my family before "Surgery Day." We had a great time but in the back of my mind the whole time was on the mass in my neck, the surgery and the treatments that awaited me.

My mother, Joanne, and her husband, Gerald, my brother, David, my sister, Rene, and her daughter, Kristen, all came up to be with me in January for the big day of the operation. It

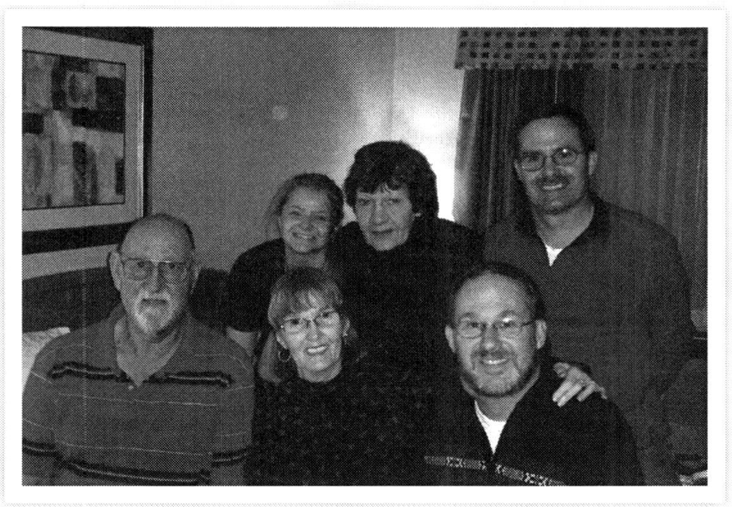

I was blessed to have my family with me, and for Debbie also, for strength in numbers.

◆　◆　◆

was nice to have them there in Madison. I treated the whole gang to what I called the "last meal" (you never know), plus I knew that pretty soon, I would not be able to eat much anyway. So we ate. It sure wasn't the best, but we ate and most of all, we enjoyed each other's company.

After our "award-winning" dinner, I took Debbie, my sister, brother, and niece on a hike to the hospital over the tracks and up the hill to those massive front doors. I walked through those front doors that night with fear, excitement and every other emotion you can think of, and up to the floor where the surgery would be performed. It was all for me. I was walking my "green mile," living the process, seeing the room, mentally preparing myself for the next day with my "cancer-fighting team." I was ready to climb my mountain in life, and that mountain got bigger as we got closer, just as they all do. And, lest we forget, it was Wisconsin in January, a nice, cold evening down into the low 20s and windy, just what my family from Arkansas needed to experience for a change.

Symbolically, I had also purchased new tennis shoes for the process and was ready to climb. We all have mountains to climb, not always by choice, but never ready to give up and give into this big ugly cancer thing. No, not me. I was wearing my big "N" on my chest, which stood for "Never give up."

Hemingway said it right:

If the world is not the enemy, neither is it our friend. In the end, no matter who surrounds us, we travel alone. Our friends and loved ones are there, providing an infrastructure of love and support. But courage must be drawn from within. Let the world see us as we see ourselves and have the faith to permit us do it our way.

During the marathon of appointments and check-ups, I remember warning the surgeon that my jugular vein and main artery were close to that large, cancer-filled lump in my neck. I'm not sure what he thought about me and my attitude, but my attitude was right for me. I've always been outspoken, and when it came to cutting on me, it was time for me to speak up in a humorous way. Humor and a positive attitude have always been at my side to help work through any tough times. This doesn't necessarily mean laughing or taking something lightly, but accepting the experience with a positive attitude.

The big day—January 27, 2009—finally came. The operating room was running about an hour late, but that was okay with me. While in the waiting area with Debbie and my entire family and God by my side, I was safe.

Three hours later, I woke up in my room in the ICU area with some nurse in a white uniform trying to push a plate of meatloaf, potatoes, and green beans in my face. Like I was supposed to eat that stuff! I was alive and on some good pain killers. That first night, they even let me push the button if I needed more pain-killing juice to help me sleep. The surgery was done; now for the treatments.

◆ ◆ ◆

The Feeding Tube People
(that's what I called them—not to their face or anything!)

Yes, you read it right, that's what I called them, the "feeding tube" people. Those were the experts knew just what I needed when I didn't. This was the process that scared me the most upfront when it came to the whole treatment process. Thinking of this thing hanging out of my stomach, wondering what do I do if it falls out or in?

The "Feeding Tube" people were right on. By the time I hit week four of radiation treatments, I wonder today what would have come of me without the ability to let that thing suck in all that awful Ensure®. By week five I was up to six plus bottles a day; this was my food, my strength, my mission every day. It kept me alive and I'm sure of it today.

If I had to coach anyone who is going through head and neck cancer with radiation in the neck or throat area, I would

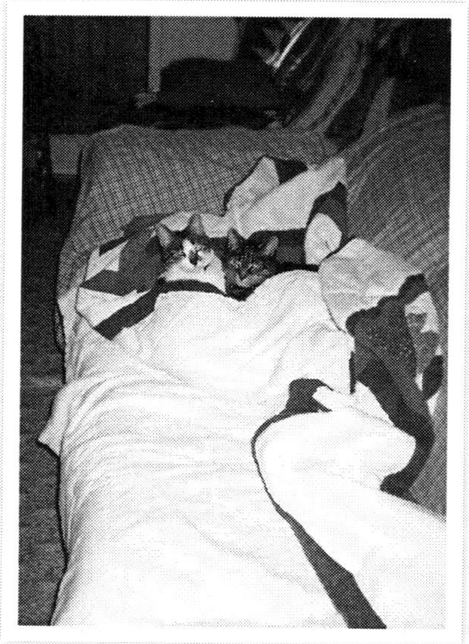

highly recommend listening and trusting your oncology team. My recommendation is get home from treatments if you can or in your room, hook it up and pour the Ensure® and lie back and watch TV, the older the shows the better, then nap a little. I was blessed to have part of my "cancer-fighting team" daily with me on the couch, Whitey and his girlfriend Peewee, my kids (cats). Every day they would relax with me and cheer me on!

One of the toughest meetings for me was the one where we discussed the feeding tube and why it was necessary. I was really worried about the gastrostomy, or surgically putting a tube through my skin and stomach wall, directly into my stomach, so that I would be able to feed myself with liquid protein. It would involve an overnight-stay surgery. But more than the insertion itself was the fear of what if it popped out! What would I do then, over two hours away from the hospital (UW–Madison) that inserted this machine (thing). I had to let that fear go and follow the recommendations. It was not about me at that time; it was about doing whatever I had to do to complete the process of ridding my body and my life of the cancer.

The feeding tube was inserted on March 19, 2009. This was beginning to be one interesting journey! When I awoke the next morning, there was this tube with a little on-and-off switch hanging out of my stomach. Before Debbie and I checked out, one of the nurses went over the process pretty quickly on how to clean it out daily, shut it on and off, and take it out to clean around it. My head was spinning and the clock had started ticking. I had about eight weeks to recover from the surgery and would then begin the thirty radiation treatments and chemotherapy sessions.

At first, the treatments were the scariest part of the process for me. They were more frightening than the surgery, for they were the unknown, the "what if," the "Can I do it?" the "What will they do to me?" the "Will I lose all my hair?" To tell you the truth, I was more worried about that than anything else. Why? Our hair defines us, and if we lose our hair, we lose a part of our identity. I like my hair. If I lose my hair, people will know something's wrong. Oh, my God, what will I do? I decided: "I will keep living with less hair." As it turned out, the radiation and chemo didn't make me lose all my hair to the degree that I looked strange to others. Keeping most of my hair was an indication to me that I was walking through the treatments. I was moving forward.

I had my new tennis shoes on, ready to fight the battle and run my race. Throughout the years, I've had many races to run, battles to fight, as do many of you. I've found that we all have a race to run, a battle or a mountain to climb. Each day, my battle with cancer brought a new challenge of some type.

◆ ◆ ◆

Post-Surgery Treatments

If you haven't guessed by now, "Never give up" is my motto. My initial plan was to drive the four-hour round trip from home, Cedarburg to Madison, every day for my radiation treatments for the next six and a half weeks. I would stay overnight in Madison the days I had my chemo treatments, rest, and drive back after radiation treatment the following morning. Easy at first, no problem, until week four of treatments. Then, the ride got tougher.

At the three-week mark of radiation treatments, I remember telling my radiation doctor that things weren't as bad as I thought they would be. I also remember him very clearly telling me to just wait until week four and the following weeks after treatment. And boy, was he right! The compounding effect of the treatments can really kick your butt!

Radiation

On Day 1 of radiation treatment, March 9, 2009, I walked in strong and standing tall as my mother always told me to do. On Treatment Day 30, my last day, April 17, 2009, I walked out as weak as a puppy and feeling all beaten up. I realized my journey had just begun!

The oncology team had explained to me that I would not be able to drive the four hours each day for 30 treatments. But I am not a quitter. I couldn't let this thing beat me, and had to prove to myself that I could get through it. I had to stay strong. Every day, from March 9 through April 17, 2009, I drove back and forth for my treatments. Every day, I would listen to my inspirational tapes—Jim Rohn, Joel Osteen, and John Maxwell are some of my favorites. I would think and talk with God about the day's activities.

Every day, I would get up at 5:30 a.m., knowing my purpose for the day: Clean out my feeding tube, eat something. (I was getting real tired of scrambled eggs and grits—I could have really used a change there. But what's a person to do? Eat!) Then get moving, shower, shave, dress, get in the car to make the two-hour drive to the hospital for my treatments, my therapy, my cure.

The first day in the radiation room was to get fitted for my "radiation mask," a hard, plastic thing molded exactly to my face and neck to ensure that the radiation could be focused on the specific area that needed the treatment. The mask felt very strange but as the treatments went on, it was just a part of the recovery process. I would lie on the table that moved into the radiation machine with my mask on, hands crossed on my chest.

My radiation treatments lasted about twenty five minutes once the assistants got me situated on the bed and fitted the tomography mask tightly to my face and neck. Once I was all strapped in, they would make sure I was comfortable then tell me it was time. It was like being in a tube with a medicine man dancing around my head, shaking his magical rattles and beating his magical drum, along with a continuous ringing, as the radiation machine went around my head and neck area.

Throughout the twenty-five minute radiation treatments, I kept my eyes closed—I just thought and prayed. Most of my prayers were not for me, but rather thanking God for what he had gifted me with, especially Debbie and our little family (three cats and Rocky, our sheltie dog).

About the middle of week three of radiation during a check-up I was asked how I felt and if I had any pain. There was a chart on the wall showing a pain scale from 1 to 10, with 10 being the greatest pain level. I responded by saying it wasn't as bad as I thought it would be, maybe around a 4. the oncologist was straightforward with me and told me to just wait until week four and the three to six weeks after radiation treatment. Because of the "compounding effect," there will be a difference in my pain level. I'm thinking "Thanks, just can't wait!"

I won't lie to you. By week four of the radiation treatments, there was a difference in everything from my pain level, to my ability to eat, drink and even want to talk. It was tough, the pain increased, and I felt truly exhausted, like there was nothing left to give. I felt empty and drained after the drive down, the treatments, the stress, the drive back, and then the feeding tube. I had a mission when I returned from treatments. I had a process: clean the tube out, salt and baking soda for my throat, and more pain-killing medicine. Reflecting back, I still don't know how I got the energy to cook Debbie dinner every night—I think only with love. Love can give you a deeper sense of purpose, and energy that comes from deep inside.

It was a time for me to stay strong and focused to my life mission and vision and not let it stop me in my tracks. Thank God for those new tennis shoes I got right before beginning my treatments; I was light on my feet and ready for the climb! And thank God for medication.

By week five, I was up to a daily dose of eight bottles of liquid protein through the feeding tube. I let the liquid nourish my system while I rested on the couch with my two cats, Whitey and PeeWee, there by my side, every day. Peanut, our third cat, was always near, but Whitey didn't like her too well so they needed their space or there would be trouble. Whitey and PeeWee are key members of the Cockerel Cancer-Fighting Team.

My hope for you, if you are the one going along this cancer-fighting journey, is that you walk through the pain, confusion, fear, and loneliness. I was the only one who could have experienced what I did, alone. Sure, Debbie was there and my family was close by, but I had to walk into the chemo room for therapy and sit there for three hours taking the juice—alone. I had to take those 30 radiation treatments by myself. I had to feed myself through the feeding tube for two months. Eating meals took a long time, at least two hours, chewing everything to mush, and that was with the good pain killers.

I lost 39 pounds because I couldn't eat the proper foods, it was pretty much Ensure® and eggs. In just a few months, I went from 179 pounds before surgery on January 06, 2009, to around 140 pounds on Mother's Day that same year. Losing that much weight was huge for me; I could feel it and see it. But I didn't let it stop me; I had to keep moving, proving to myself that I was bigger than this thing called cancer. It was a battle I was not going to lose.

As the weeks passed, the pain became stronger and I would pull over from my trips to and from Madison for my treatments and take a small dose of pain killer to help with my swallowing. I tried milk shakes like the oncology team had suggested, but those tasted terrible to me. One time, I even tried to eat some good, hot, and salty McDonald's fries and chicken nuggets, but those didn't go down too easily either. Nothing really tasted good from about week three of my treatments until the end of May. Friends, allow me to say, I like to eat, and for a little guy, I can eat a lot of food.

On the last day of treatment, April 17, I met with the radiation team and set my follow-up appointments. For the next four weeks, I would have weekly check-ups. I was ready to move on through the healing process from the treatments and on to conquering my dreams!

Each check-up meeting involved the radiation doctor and chemotherapy doctor, lots of blood tests, poking in my arm, hand, or wherever they could insert a needle. That got old real fast, but was part of the process I had to work through. My goal with each visit was to get through it as quickly as possible, then get home with my feeding tube, pour in some protein drink, and hang out with the cats. The best part of the day was when Debbie came home from work and I could cook her dinner. Even though I couldn't eat much of anything, it was still a joy to be doing something for someone I love.

Chemotherapy

The chemo treatments went as well as treatments can go. My chemotherapy sessions began on March 10, 2009, and every Tuesday for six weeks. Those were long days. I would leave home around 7 a.m., after cleaning out the feeding tube and using my salt-and-baking soda process and drinking down a shot or two of Oxycodine® (Roxicet), the pain-killing medicine for my throat and soul. I would arrive at the UW–Madison clinic, go right to check in for my radiation treatments, which would take place after a ten- to thirty-minute wait time.

Once I was strapped in with my radiation facemask, the radiation process would begin. After that was done, it would be off to another floor, the oncology chemotherapy area. People would be sitting in the waiting room with their IVs waiting for their time, and I joined them as soon as I checked in. The wait was quick, with thoughts of how will it go today, how will I feel tonight and what will I eat. I hated those days, but never gave up on the process.

When it was my turn and my name was called, the nurse would take me to my own special room with a comfortable recliner and a small flat-screen TV. The chemo would start with one of three bags, two with saline and one with the "poison," the chemo Cisplatin®, done intravenously. The rhythm was one water-based liquid, the chemo, and one more bag to help me cleanse my system. After the second bag, I would go to the bathroom to get all the chemo I could out of my system. If not, I would get a shot that would help me. Didn't need any more shots! The process took 3 to 3½ hours, during which I couldn't really read or concentrate. I would just sit back and listen to others and think.

After the chemo session, I would work my way down to the cafeteria to try and find something that I could eat after a full day of radiation and chemo treatments. They did have ice cream and flavorful juices, which always felt good on my throat. Then I would trundle over to a hotel close to the hospital, land my weary bones for the night and wait until the next round of radiation in the morning. What a day Tuesdays turned out to be. Maybe this is where the title, "stormy Tuesdays" or was that "stormy Mondays" came from? It was all the same to me.

I didn't like the chemotherapy—it made me feel really strange afterwards. While I didn't get really sick, I stayed in a hotel room those days and nights and didn't try to drive home. I was just too worn out, drained of any energy to speak of. On radiation treatment days, I would drive the four-hour round trip and get home and hit the couch with my four-legged Cancer-Fighting Team. Then I'd go through my process. I still managed to cook dinner for Debbie every day. This gave me purpose. I also thought if I couldn't eat well, she should eat for both of us. I would cook all the things I wished I could've eaten. I had no sense of smell or taste, other than the weird metallic taste the oncology folks had told me about.

My response to chemo treatments was, "I'm going to get through this, get to my hotel room, rest, and can't wait until the next day to get my radiation treatment done and get home." I could have reacted to the chemotherapy with bad thoughts, which could have resulted in negative physical reactions. But I chose not to.

Please don't get me wrong. Therapy was not a happy time at all. It was a scary time, an uncomfortable time; more worry about the "what ifs…" than anything. Chemotherapy or radiation treatments aren't what we dream about as being our deepest desires and dreams, but in most cases, they are related to cancer treatment. And they were what I had to do to fight my battle. My motto: "It is what it is"!

◆　◆　◆

Life After Treatments
Rebuilding The Mind, The Body, And The Soul

I might be putting the cart before the horse early in the book talking about life after treatments, but I need to get you there. The treatments were somewhat like a challenge to me: getting through them became not just a task, but a mission and my purpose.

My positive attitude was my medicine and I knew I had to battle the odds at all cost. Today, those treatments are behind me, but the memories are still there. I can reflect and feel those sensations at times; it's scary wondering if I ever will be faced with the whole enchilada again.

While writing this book, I am in the rebuilding season of my life, getting my weight back up to around 169 (it's currently at 154 and climbing), eating all the good stuff I can, taking care of my body, and knowing I need to work out more often. My profession as a trainer puts me on the road five days a week, with 10 to 14 hours a day training and doing business coaching. My mind is as strong as it was throughout the process. My spirit is getting stronger and deeper in faith. I really believe that there has to be someone bigger, greater who has helped me along this journey.

Debbie retired on December 31, 2009, which was a goal we had been working toward for a while—we have too many things to do together. I can't and won't let this thing called cancer win. We have more vacations to take and more places to go. I want to retire and live the easy life. I have more books to read and more to write, more speeches to share and stories to tell. My mind is strong and the mind controls the body. I must keep moving and looking forward. I know that this thing can take over me if it wants to. I know in many cases it wins; today is just not the day.

◆ ◆ ◆

Back To The Intention Of This Book

My purpose in sharing my journey with you is to offer encouragement and hope. I believe the "Big C" can stand for more than "Cancer." It can stand for "Cure" or "Change," which is what we have to do to keep enjoying our gift of life. I also believe that **C.A.N.C.E.R.** can give you six reasons to keep living and enjoying your gift of life. As you read on, I hope my own story will help you along your journey through cancer, or that of a loved one or friend. I hope and pray that you can find that "bigger thing" in your life that makes the inexplicable happen. Faith can help you in this area, and my sincere wish for you is that you will find a way to enjoy the journey as I have, and will keep living to give.

For me, the acronym **C.A.N.C.E.R.** stands for good, not evil; hope, not despair; faith, not fear, companionship, not loneliness; cure, not death; encouragement, not discouragement; healing, not fading; giving, not taking; loving, not hating; believing, not forgetting. My hope for you is that you or a loved one gets better, first mentally, psychologically, spiritually, and then physically.

The words I lived by along my journey, and still do, are:

C	Conquer Your Dreams
A	Attitude is Everything
N	Never Give Up
C	Change is Okay
E	Encourage Others
R	Reflect and Grow

Follow my lead and you may find that this thing called **C.A.N.C.E.R.** can be a friend, if you allow it. I've found that it's an attitude, a choice; do I let it beat me down or fight the battle? My final answer to this question is, fight the battle!

C.A.N.C.E.R. can help you keep living and enjoying your gift of life!

a snapshot from my journey

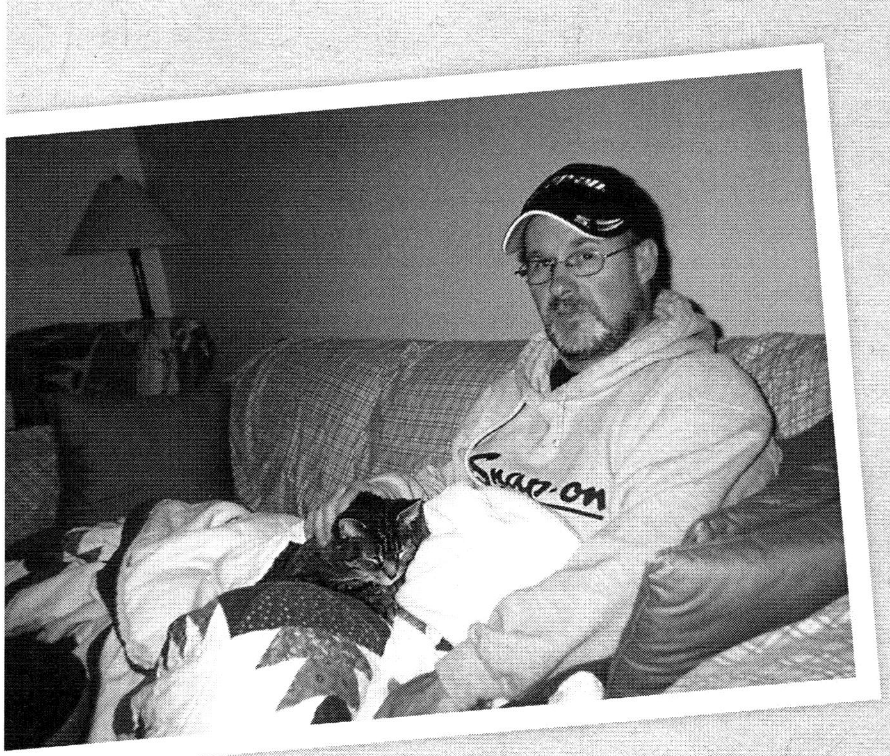

PeeWee, one of my cancer-fighting team members, and me, in February 2009 after surgery, resting and waiting for my treatments, which started March 9, 2009.

◆ ◆ ◆

I found it takes a very special team to fight the good fight for life; family, pets, surgeons, chemotherapy and radiation specialists, the "feeding tube people" (that's what I called them) and most of all, Debbie, my best friend and life partner.

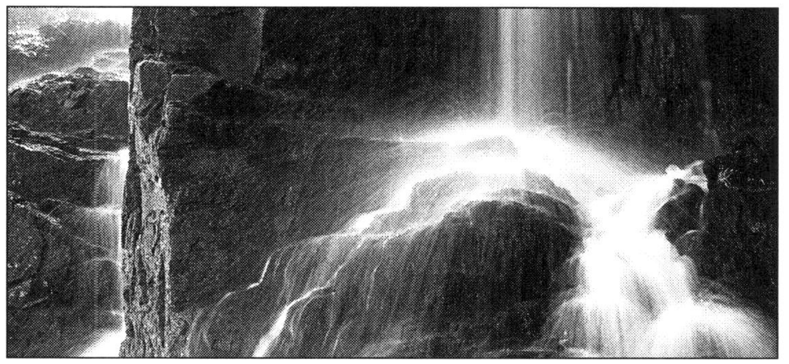

The journey is full of life's gifts—

conquer your dreams

...The meaning of life, the journey

Everyone hopes to discover the meaning of life. What is your mission, your purpose, and your meaning for the life you have been gifted? We all search daily for the answers. We pray, read, seek guidance, and even travel the world searching for meaning.

The true question is: Is what we're searching for awaiting within us?

Do we hold all the answers?

We hear about those who come through the worst situations and continue to live their lives giving to others. We know of those who have more than they would ever know what to do with. There are multi-billionaires, people with more money than some of us can even imagine. Then there are those less fortunate who are still able to spend their lives helping others in far-away countries.

I've asked myself the "purpose and meaning" questions many times over the years. There have been multiple answers, depending on what season of life I was in, who was in my life, and where I was along my journey. I've come to think that the answer was tied to where I was in my life. Today, my meaning of life is to find ways to return, give, and offer hope and encouragement.

In 1975, I attempted suicide, which was a scream for help and search for self-identity. In 1984, my meaning of life was to climb the corporate ladder. In 1985, it was to survive a terrible accident. In 1990, my mission was to get married and be a husband. By 2000, my meaning of life was to develop a business and to add value to business professionals. In 2009, it was to expand my business, add value to leaders and make a difference in the lives of teens. From 2010 on, my purpose and meaning of life has become sharing my cancer story and encouraging hope.

My meaning of life is always evolving. My journey takes me to new places daily, new ways to grow and learn. My gift of life is about giving and making a difference in the lives of others by sharing the experiences that have made an impact in my life. Looking back today, the cancer diagnosis could have been a negative experience; it has turned out to be positive at many different levels. I learned so much about myself, recognized my strong drive to survive, and today, my most sincere desire is to use this experience to positively impact the lives of others in whatever way I can.

What about your life? Can all the challenges and opportunities you've experienced be considered hope, inspiration, or a lesson learned that another could grow from?

The journey is what we make it, and how we think about the situations, events, and outcomes. Life is a series of making choices; how we choose to react or respond to life's events can make the difference in how we live our gift of life.

I had many choices. React or respond? To respond is to take responsibility for one's mental and emotional state, to stay in control. Reacting puts control in someone or something else's court. How did I react or respond to the information coming at me like a freight train in the fall of 2008? How did I react or respond to all those tests, biopsies, and recommendations? I learned quickly to respond. When under pressure, fear, and confusion, it's always best to respond, to look at things from a place of choice. To tell the truth, though, there were certainly a few times this guy who had never been sick in his life reacted. Mostly it was out of fear of the "unknown," the "what ifs..." that cancer offers.

My message to you is about discovering or re-discovering your meaning of life, your purpose, your ability to respond and not react to your cancer. I hope the words in this little book will help you resolve to be a fighter and stay positive while fighting the good battle of life.

I have chosen to turn my gift of life into a gift of hope and encouragement, rather than leaving it in the closet with the rest of the stuff I brought back from the hospital as souvenirs. My friends, I have decided to write and share my story, from a speaker's platform, from the pages of this book. I want more than anything else to do something good with my gift. That's my choice. I could of sat back and consumed my life with all the negatives that cancer brings and live in that mind set, or make the choice to not live in it, but work through it. I still have many dreams to conquer, many, many things to do and achieve. I'm not ready to live out my "bucket list" today, but live out my "life list," the things I can do daily to live my life to its fullest potential.

What about you?

Allow me to share a very important thought with you: you should not be satisfied with being a victim of cancer, or with being just a survivor. I recommend that you set your sights on being a conqueror. I've found that there is this extraordinary quality of spirit that leads one to aspire to conquering dreams rather than just surviving. I believe that we are either evolving or existing. I just don't want to exist, I want to live, be success-ful, happy, content in my life with Debbie.

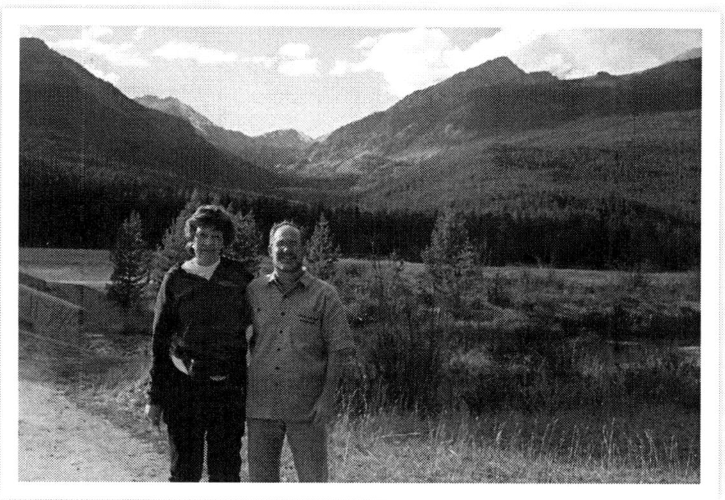

I am conquering my dreams every day that I can share and enjoy my life with Debbie. Rocky Mountain National Park in October 2007 where I first noticed the lump on my neck.

I'm aggressively living my life every day by sharing, laughing, and living to give.

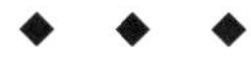

The "BIG C" could have a lot more meanings than just "cancer." In my message to you today, it means "conquer your dreams"!

The letter "C" was a good grade for me during my school years. The letter "C" can also stand for C-Class Executives in Corporate America. It can also stand for "Cure," meaning there is hope.

Choose to conquer your dreams. The journey is full of life's gifts, and these gifts are our dreams coming true: the dream of getting a good job out of high school or college, the dream of marriage, the dream of owning your own home or business, to having children, grandchildren, and retirement.

Dreams come true every day. You might dream of walking again, of feeling love again, of holding a loved one again. Hold onto the dream to keep living and beating your cancer. The dream I held onto while I went through the radiation and chemotherapy treatments was eating all the food I wished I could have eaten during treatments. And friends, I did!

Life is good, no matter how bad it gets at times, no matter how rough the treatments are. There is hope, hope for tomorrow, hope for a cure, and hope for a way to make a difference.

Life is full of gifts, some wrapped with a pretty bow, others in a box, a chemo bag, an x-ray machine, or a medicine bottle. Once you have the gift, what do you do with it? Yes, I see my cancer as a gift, a gift to be shared and just one of life's weird little gifts, like a white elephant present, that in some cases, we can do good with. I made a decision to look at this awful subject (cancer) as a gift, not a disease, not as evil, but as one of my life gifts that I'm supposed to do something good with.

I can't pass the cancer along and wouldn't if I could, but I can pass along inspiration, hope, and encouragement from my cancer experience. My mission today is to offer hope and encouragement to everyone I meet. You can't pass it along, or drop it off at the next corner. Once cancer has you, you've got to do something with it. You can let it eat you up or take over your life, or not.

During my three-hour chemotherapy treatments, I met two ladies in the therapy room across from mine who were planning their Hawaiian trip. One was "taking the poison," the other, her partner or friend, was there for support. Their plan was in action: how would they handle the medication, what would they eat, where would they go, and what would they see? While listening to and then talking with them, I understood their mission and purpose. They were planning their last big vacation. They were conquering their dreams, together. I just knew they were not going to let anything— and I mean anything—stand in their way.

I've found that cancer is a path you must travel alone at times, but without love and friends and family, it can be a very lonely journey. The gift of a friend, mate, or family member by your side during your journey is like a gift from heaven, like an angel in my eyes.

One song I listened to frequently on my drive between Cedarburg and Madison for my daily treatments was Tim McGraw's *Live Like You Were Dying*. I truly believe this concept should be carried out more often by more people, even those without cancer or some other life-threatening illness. Learn to live life to your fullest potential each and every day, no excuses!

Conquering my dreams is my personal mission. My dream is to give, to inspire, to motivate change, and to serve the growth of others. My dream is not working five days a week the rest of my life. My dream is to spend more time with

Debbie, read more, speak more, and coach and train more sales professionals and business professionals on how to maximize their potential. My dream is to reach out to others with cancer and offer hope, permission to keep living and enjoying life, and not to give in or give up.

One of my dreams is to take Debbie on as many cool vacations and places we've never been, to experience things we haven't experienced. One of these vacations has to be on a beach with the sun shining and those awesome little drinks with umbrellas in them. No cold, no snow. That trip will need to be right in the middle of one of our Wisconsin winters. No rushing around, no loud noises, just a slow, easy, relaxing vacation. Friends, let me tell you this will happen. That dream will become reality. Already, our life journey together has taken us many places and will take us many more new places; there is no real destination, it's in the journey.

Life's journey is not a destination. Success is not a destination. There isn't a final depot or drop-off place. Life's journey is a process of connecting with others, making decisions, fulfilling dreams, impacting others, changing lives, offering hope, and enjoying life with your loved ones. This life is good, and I can't wait to see what awaits me: I know there must be something bigger, better, and even more fulfilling to discover.

Remember, the "C" stands for "Conquer your Dreams." Don't let anything get in your way. You need to pay the cost, take the risk, and make the decisions that will move you closer daily to your dream fulfillment.

Your journey is full of life's gifts just waiting for you. Life is a gift. Some call it a "present." The ability to live in the present and not the past or in the future allows you to deal with the present. Either we are regretting something in the past that we cannot change, or we are worrying about something in the future that our worry is going to bring about. Live in today and you can live in joy and make the future what you envision.

Conquer your dreams! It's about you—not the cancer.

a snapshot from my journey

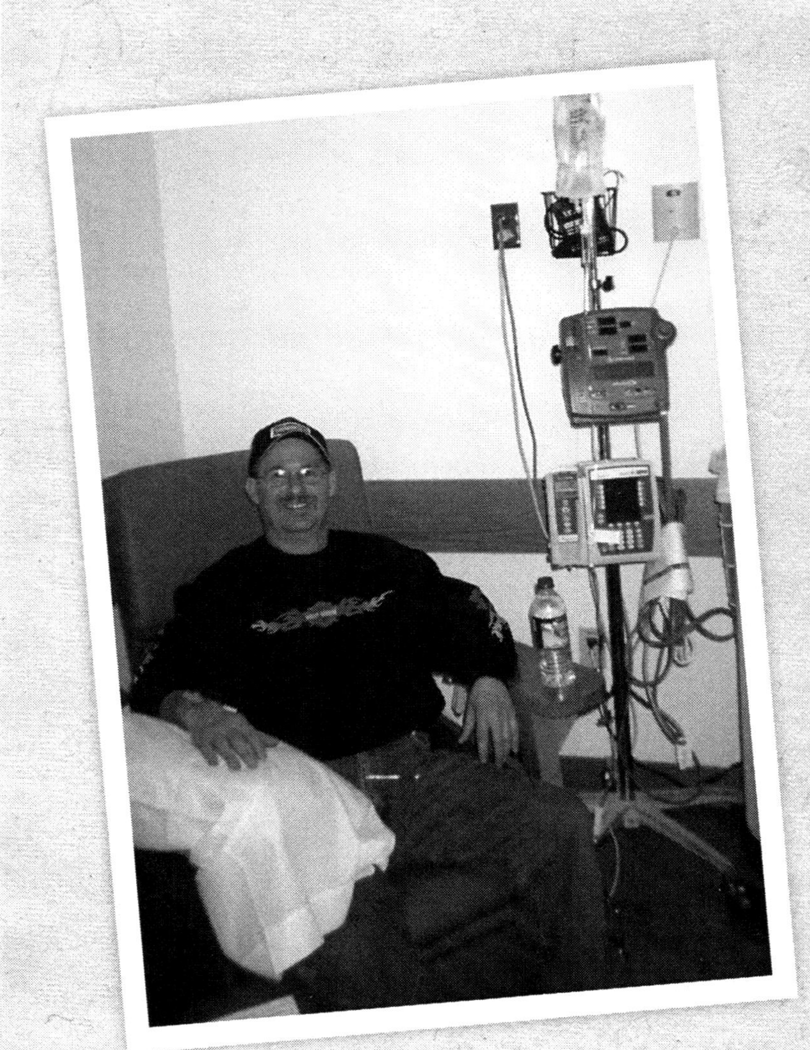

Attitude is everything when it comes to chemo day.

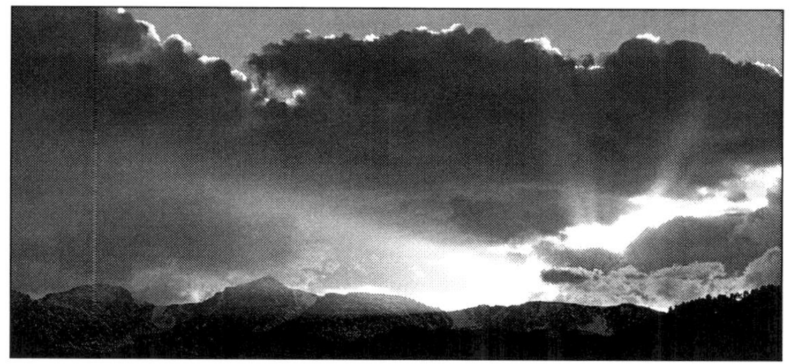

Battling the odds at all cost—
attitude is everything

...Life after treatments.
Rebuilding the mind, body, & soul

Chemo day was all about attitude and having a good attitude about a very terrifying subject. Let me tell you, I sat there with a smile on my face because I was alive, but I was also scared to death. I'd only heard negative things about chemotherapy, nothing good. I watched my dad go through chemotherapy back in the 1980s with lung cancer, to Debbie's dad (Ed) chemotherapy with pancreatic cancer in 2005 and her sister (Susy) and her chemotherapy a couple of years later with colon cancer treatments. My first treatment was not fun at all. Later that night, I sat there not knowing what was going to happen afterwards or that night in my hotel room. After my treatment, I would go through my process in the hotel room.

Attitude was my four-leaf clover; I had to keep a positive attitude about my decision to take on the treatments and keep moving forward, not knowing what awaited me. Those nights after chemo were hard: cold chills throughout the night, nausea, and fear of the unknown.

Attitude—the way we look at life, the way we handle change, and the way we respond to others—is everything. Cancer is scary, fearful, mean, and ugly. It wears a face no one wants to mirror, lives a life many don't understand. Millions of dollars are spent annually on research for a cure of all the many types of cancers. Battling the odds is doing whatever you have to do to keep focused on getting better, getting through your treatments, and adapting to your new life.

Attitude is the key to your recovery, to an exciting future picture, to your relationships, and your ability to manage your treatments. A positive attitude may not get you everything in life, but it will take you more places than a negative attitude. Keep the faith with respect to your positive attitude about your cancer, your journey, and your ability to fight the good fight of faith.

When fighting cancer, keep your focus on your treatments and lift your attitude about the process you have to go through. I'm not trying to make this sound easy. You have a long, tough road ahead of you. It's not an easy fight. The path is long and hard, and the mental stress and body changes are difficult. The sickness and weakness, the pain, the heartbreak, the potential loss of a fellow traveler— it's all real hard.

But what are we supposed to do? Stop fighting, give in, lie down, and quit? An emphatic "NO!" Keep fighting, battle the odds at all costs, and take the risk with new medications or new treatments. Don't let anyone say you have six months, or two years, or however long they might predict. They are not in control of your life—you are!

Keep in mind that attitude is also everything for your loved ones, your friends, associates, and others who are watching to see how you deal with your cancer, the ugly beast. The mountain is meant to be climbed, the journey is meant to be lived and shared, and the battle is meant to be fought together.

The longer you live, the more you may realize the impact of your attitude on life. I'm convinced that life is ten percent what happens to you and ninety percent how you respond to it. Our attitude is the one thing we can control.

Even though some folks might scoff at the idea of a positive attitude, I say, "Let's compare it to a negative attitude and what that will do for you." I've found no matter what's happening in my life, whether it was a promotion that didn't come my way or a lotto ticket that said "Not a Winner," I've still kept a positive perspective, a good attitude, and everything seemed to just work out. I tell myself, "Maybe next time," and purchase another ticket! I think it's likely that if the grumpies or grumbles had worked their way in, things would have not worked out as well. Never give up, right?

My Attitude About Cost

Let's look at the words, "whatever it costs." Ask yourself if it's worth whatever it takes? Yes! Your life and those who you love and those who love you are worth the cost, whatever the cost.

At all cost, keep moving forward and giving it all you got. Stay open to your ideas and dreams. Don't lie down and quit; keep thinking about tomorrow and what you have to live for. Remember the friends and family members who are in your corner, as well as all the research teams working on a cure. No one has given up. Don't you!

Life is all about the costs. You've got to pay to play. There is always a cost to fight; the good fight for life is worth it. Don't give up or give in, friends. Fight the good fight with faith, hope, and love. Don't let the giant win; you don't have to fight the battle alone. God is always there. Others are close.

I love paying the cost. Here are a few examples: I love paying the cost of being a Harley dude, with the leathers and the chrome. I love paying the cost of learning to play the guitar; a couple of really cool guitars will set you back a few hundred to a few thousand. I love paying the cost of creating a good, comfortable life for Debbie and me. I love paying the cost of traveling for my business, sleeping in hotels, not eating as well as I should—a life on the road has been my lifestyle for many years. Truthfully, I look forward to slowing down, working less, and living more. When you pay the cost for those things that truly bring joy, the costs aren't as big as the rewards.

When I was told that I had cancer, I knew there would be costs: time, money, and more. The costs I was willing to pay had no price tag. I would do whatever I had to do. I've found over the years that the cost that must be paid for change is critical to getting what you want out of life. Nothing good comes easy. There are always costs to pay, the cost of your time away from your family, the cost to change is the fear of the unknown. I would do whatever it took, things I would have ever thought about doing, knowing nothing about. Whatever the cost, I was ready to pay to deal with my cancer and rid it from my body and my life to the best of my ability.

I don't know where to start when it comes to sharing my story regarding the expenses involved. The expenses were huge: the treatments, the appointments, the medication, the fuel to get to and from appointments—all told, $200,000+ over a six-month period. I'm just lucky to have had good insurance. As a self-employed speaker and trainer, I pay highly for that coverage. What would I have done if I hadn't had insurance coverage or a good plan that paid for almost 95% of all my expenses to date? I would have made the same choices and done the same things.

Without the surgery and treatments, my life could have been over in two to five years.

Good health insurance helps, but no insurance can make it tough. I'm to believe there are resources available to those without coverage.

My expenses haven't gotten lower and my insurance premiums have soared from $245 to well over $600 per month, but it's a cost I must pay. I'm writing to offer hope and encouragement through this very challenging and difficult time. We spent more in six months then we paid for our home in Cedarburg, Wisconsin, when we bought it. The cost question again: Am I willing to pay the cost to stay alive, to fight the battle, to survive and thrive? A resounding "Yes"!

My Attitude About Change

Change is scary, uncomfortable, and when it came to cancer, I knew I would have to change my lifestyle, as well as my attitude about doctors and medicine. I told myself that no matter what I thought, read, or heard from others, it was time to step up and change my thinking, to open my mind and trust in others.

When I encounter change, I do my best to view it as a good opportunity to learn, grow, and invest in my future, my vision, and my mission.

When something comes your way and change is on the horizon, are you willing to change, change that will lift you, alter you, and make you a better person? I am. I have to believe that cancer has helped me change my outlook on life, my relationships, and my purpose all in a good way. Change is okay!

Negative thoughts can give a negative return. It's always better to keep a positive attitude. Hang on to the good thoughts about your progression to a better you. Cancer has taught me that I have new choices in life, the choice of life over death. Cancer has been a good teacher with respect to what I do with my time and my life. Through my cancer, I've discovered that new choices means new experiences and opportunities to add value to others.

Change Means Choice

I had a choice. I could allow fear to settle in: fear of the surgery, fear of the feeding tube, the treatments, and the chemo. Fear of what if it doesn't work after it's all said and done? Or I could choose to allow new-found courage, faith, and ability to accept the cancer, accept the treatments as a cost of wellness, and the courage to keep living and enjoying my gift of life.

Think about the choices we make every day: what to eat, what to wear, do I get that new flat-screen TV or do I invest in more books to read and places to go? Life is a continuous flow of choices and it's what we do with those choices that makes the differences in our life and the lives of others.

I made the conscious choice to follow the doctors' lead, do whatever they suggested, and get up and drive to my treatments every day, even though I was told I wouldn't be able to keep it up. My choice was to live.

◆　◆　◆

Your Attitude Determines Your Self-Worth, Which Can Determine Your Net Worth!

Life is full of obstacles that allow us to grow, learn, and expand our thinking. Is the battle ever over? No. I've learned and accepted that once one hill has been climbed, it allowed me to see other hills to climb. After each climb, my hope was to get smarter and better, maybe more adaptable, flexible, and faithful for another day's climb. Through this cancer battle, I've learned to be more thoughtful, thankful, and faithful. In fact, the cancer journey has been like a mentor or teacher, helping me appreciate what I've been blessed with and how much my family means to me, far more than money or things. Hanging on to those teachings helped me maintain my positive attitude.

Not only did the cancer fill my life with fear and uncertainty, it also opened my eyes to what people and things are really important in the short time we have on earth. The cancer helped me see the beauty in things I'd never really spent time with before. Things like just taking it easy at home, not always being on the move, and reading. Over the past few years, I've wanted to read and expand my thinking and grow. I really enjoy my thinking time more in my life now than ever before, just nice clear, quiet thinking time. I believe that when you're faced with something that is bigger than you are, the unknown or fears, your perspective of life changes.

You've heard the phrases, "Life's too short... Live one day at a time." Life is precious; time is our gift to share with others, loved ones. It truly is the little things in life that can make the biggest differences.

I'm a much more thankful person today. I've learned quickly to appreciate others who have cancer and other illnesses and the battles that they may be facing, the fears, the worry, the unknown. I've also learned to be more thoughtful of others and to my time and health. I've developed a deeper passion for others that honestly wasn't there prior to my experience.

Like you, I have a choice of either looking at only the bad things that could occur, or learning to look for the good things that could help me grow and be a better person. To me, it really was all good stuff, positive things that have come out of the cancer journey. When you look with a positive attitude, you can always find good in what is bad. It just means opening your eyes and seeking the good.

You've also likely heard, "Anything free is just about as good as what you paid for it: nothing!" I'm not sure that applies to everything, though. Love is free—or is it? There is a big cost to pay in love, your feelings, emotional state, the cost of trust and faith in your partner. The cost isn't always in dollars, but within your heart. If things don't go so well, love hurts. That's the cost I'm talking about. But when love is good, life is great. I've personally found that the rewards are greater than any financial investment that can be made: the reward in good relationships, love and trust I think is the most powerful motivator to help you get through anything.

When you are faced with cancer or another illness or challenge, remember that it's your life, not that of the cancer or the other problems or illnesses. It's your body. You own the body God gifted you with, along with the mind, soul, and power to fight the evil. Be strong, my friend. If there is hope in the future, there is power in the now. Live your life thankfully, thoughtfully, and faithfully. Enjoy the ride, even when you hit the bumps, the walls, and the sharp turns. You are a warrior, fighting the good fight for your life—no matter what it costs.

I pray that you will discover the power of a positive attitude within you and continue to fight the good fight, no matter what it costs. We have one life to live; it's our duty to ourselves and our loved ones to fight our best fight, and climb our mountain to achieve victory. Giving it all you have, no matter how rough the road gets is what living your best life is all about, with or without cancer.

Let me tell you in the beginning days of this journey, it was scary. No, frightening. And all the talk about what if it's cancer, surgery, radiation, and the worst one, chemo. That word alone can have you shaking in your boots. The stress levels went through the roof, not only for me but also for Debbie. This thing came at us like a runaway train.

From the first meeting with the first physician to the needle biopsies, to the wrong diagnosis, it was hard on the soul. This thing can be like an unwanted earthquake shaking your life up. It was for us, and the journey was just beginning.

a snapshot from my journey

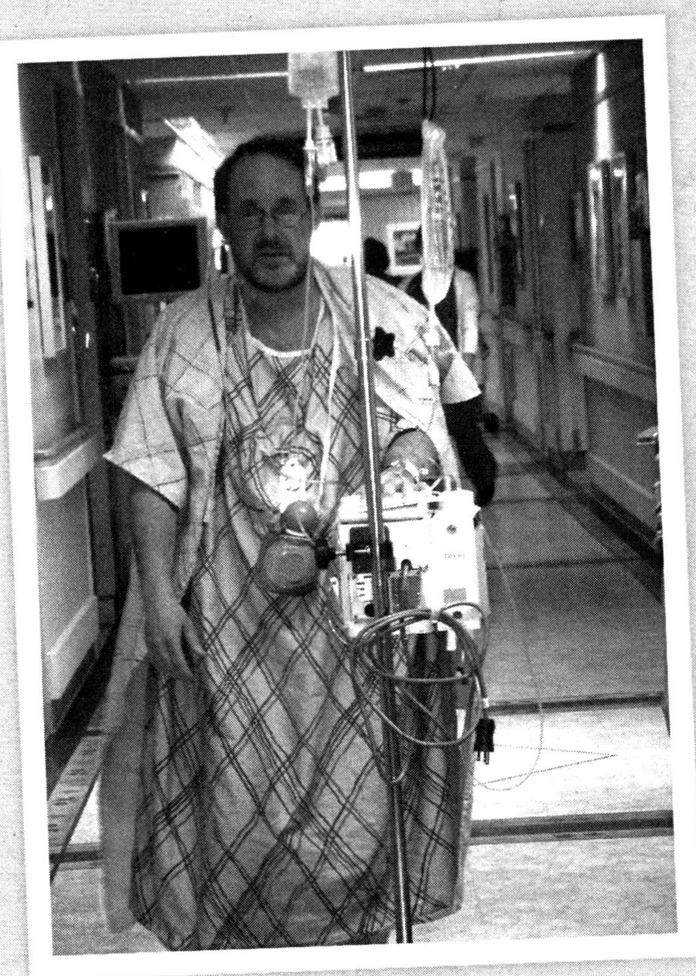

Never give up. Here I am walking the night after surgery.

reason three

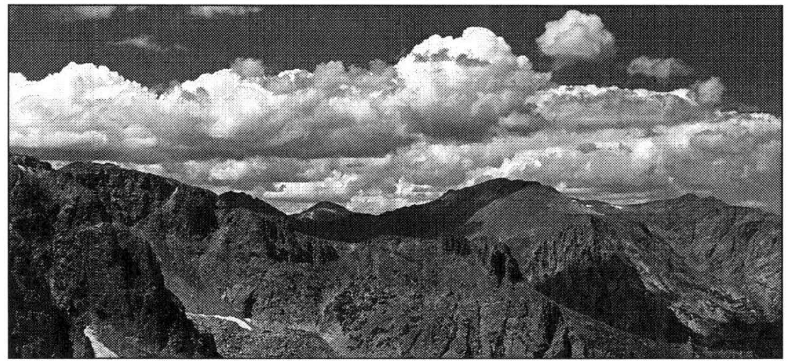

We all have a mountain to climb—

never give up

...What appears to be big, gets even bigger

My surgery day was a big day for me, the beginning of my recovery process and eliminating cancer from my body. This day was hard on me, scary and fearful of what if something goes wrong, what if I don't come out of it? Even though I had the best surgeon on the project, the best medical team at UW–Madison, my family by my side, and God with me in the operating room, I was scared to death. I'm not lying. I was afraid for Debbie, our life together, our four kids (pets) at home, and our future. In my heart, I was ready, ready to do whatever it took not to die, not to give up, to live and keep living, not just for me, but for Debbie and my family there by my side that day.

I was not going to give up or give into cancer. My surgery day was my first step to fight my battle, to kick butt on my cancer and to prove to myself that I was ready for the journey. I love Debbie and our lives together and I was not going to let my attitude go negative, or allow any fears to slow me down and stop me from doing whatever I had to do to cleanse my system of cancer. Not then and not today!

My motto is "never give up" on your cancer, your self-worth your loved ones, your dreams, and your battle.

Never give up. Don't stop paying the cost, taking the chemo, the radiation, or the medication. Don't let the treatments or the pain or the discomfort or the nausea beat you. I know it's easier to say than do, as we all have different abilities and levels of acceptance, but I've found that giving up isn't the way.

The cancer mountain is big, really big. It takes a lot of courage, help, understanding, faith, and love to pull yourself up and over to the other side. Getting to the other side is not necessarily a cure-all, but it could be an accomplishment, a victory, a little win. I've found that the more victories and accomplishments I can achieve, the greater my strength and willingness to keep going and to keep living a joyful life.

One person's mountain can be taller and harder to climb than another's. What may look like a gentle hill to one person can appear as Mount Everest to someone else. Back in October 2007, when I first really noticed that the lump on my neck was growing, Debbie and I were vacationing at Pikes Peak. We rode the Harley up and walked over to the outlook, standing arm in arm on top of the huge mountain, more than 14,000 feet up. As we gazed out at the breathtaking landscape at our feet, a hiker came up a trail that coiled up the side of the mountain. He told us it had taken him six hours to climb. I remember saying to Debbie that hiking up would be a great adventure. That spectacular day, I didn't have a clue about what my future held. Looking back, I would rather have climbed the real Pikes Peak than my cancer mountain!

Life is good, God is good, and Debbie is good. Debbie's strength gave me the internal fortitude to drive four hours back and forth for treatments every day, to cook her dinner every night, and to keep climbing my mountain. If I had given up, she would have been impacted tremendously. I'm not saying to live your life for others, but it's okay to live for others; they live their life for you. There is amazing power in having a friend, a loved one, someone by your side, willing and able to climb with you, no questions asked.

What is cancer good for? It helps you climb the mountains in your life.

Allow me to share with you 20 things about my mountain:

- My mountain helped challenge me, change me, and make me a better person.

- My mountain taught me to slow down.

- My mountain forced me to make decisions, climb higher, and give more freely.

- My mountain helped me to see things differently.

- My mountain taught me to accept things that I could not change.

- My mountain helped me to love more deeply than I have ever loved before.

- My mountain helped me to be more thankful for what I have.

- My mountain helped me to be more thoughtful towards others than ever before.

- My mountain helped me to be more faithful.

- My mountain caused me to reflect and appreciate life more.

- My mountain helped me to know myself better.

- My mountain forced me to deal with what I didn't understand.

- My mountain helped me face the unknown without fear.

- My mountain taught me that cancer can't beat me or win me over.

- ◆ My mountain showed me that I can climb higher in life.

- ◆ My mountain gave me a new perspective about life and my mission.

- ◆ My mountain took me to new heights so I could see a new vision for my life.

- ◆ My mountain is mine to climb, just like your mountain belongs to you.

- ◆ My mountain helped me answer the cost question and know that I was willing to pay whatever it took—in time, money, energy, whatever.

- ◆ My mountain's name is Larry—not "cancer," not "illness." It's just a good ol' mountain called Larry.

I could have shared 20 things the mountain did to me; instead, I chose to look at all the things the climb helped me be, and see, and do. What gifts has your mountain given you?

Take some time with a pen and paper and write out what your mountain has given to you. Learn to appreciate the mountain, not hate the climb. Don't be afraid. I write to you to offer you encouragement and hope for a good life, a joyful and thankful life.

You can choose to help others with your journey. You can lead the way to hope for another, as I hope I am doing with this little book.

Researchers claim that one out of every three people you meet will either have had some form of cancer or know someone with cancer. Recognize all those opportunities to share your mountain with others.

I would not wish cancer or any other sickness on my worst enemy, but I would wish to offer my gift of cancer as hope and encouragement to anyone who has or knows someone with cancer. I've found that my life is supposed to be lived for others. All my experiences, wins, and losses are to be experiences that can offer hope, change, recommendations, and encouragement or motivation to others. We know that we come and we go; it's what we do with this gift of life that makes the difference along the way.

Make your mountain yours. Make it big and climb to the top and enjoy the view. Take the climb at your own pace. Don't give up along the way. The view can be great, depending on how we choose to see things. Make the right choices, keep a clean mind, look for the good, praise the good. Be thankful, not dreadful; be thoughtful, not shameful; be faithful, not fearful. Living your life faithfully, thankfully, and thoughtfully can make a difference along your journey, as well as throughout the climb.

It's your mountain, your life, and your cancer. You manage as you will. Just please remember, it's all in the choices you make that will make you. Good hiking to you. Climb the tallest mountain you can find, reach the top, and be joyful you made it. Look out over your life and know you're blessed and watched after. God loves you and you had better love yourself as well. You don't have to love the disease that's in you, or what it's done to you, or may do to you, but you are still here and there and everywhere.

The Harder You Push Yourself, The Farther You Realize You Can Go

Whether you have cancer or any illness, or are perfectly healthy, follow your heart. Your time is limited, so don't waste it living someone else's life.

This thing (cancer) can take over your hours and days, run your life, consume your world, and make you believe it's in control—if you allow it to. It can define who you are, where you're going, and the timetable of life. We can buy in to that control if we choose. The diagnosis isn't always the prognosis. The verdict can be overruled. A stay of execution can be handed down. And the mind can control the body to a certain degree.

I've had the opportunity to experience many "miracles," some may call them. I refer to them as "faith-based actions." I believe there is a God. He has worked in my life, and I believe He is working right now as I write and share with you. I know He was working the day I met Debbie, and the day I talked with Robert Ian at Taco John's.

I would think that many of my readers can think back on many times where the right person was there for you or you were there for them or where something just fell into place because someone was involved. I believe we all have experienced some form of a "miracle" in our lives at one time or another. I believe that things don't just happen, but that they happen for a reason. Either I'm doing the right thing at the right time, following my passion and purpose or just the fact that God is in control of a situation and made it His. It then works out so well that I think it's a miracle.

Let me go back to Reverend Billy Graham's book, *The Journey: Living by Faith in an Uncertain World*, which emphasizes faith in God, even when life is confusing for us. I read and studied this book throughout my therapy and afterwards. It wasn't until August 2009 when we invited my sister, Rene, up from Arkansas to visit with us and enjoy our Wine and Harvest Festival in Cedarburg that I let it go. She had seen the book and said that she liked Billy Graham. I then shared the story of why I had the book. That Sunday morning, before we took her to the airport, I wrapped the book and told her not to open the package until she got home. I gave my sister the book as a gift because it had been given to me as a gift as well.

Was the book a miracle for me? Yes, I was led to the book. It wasn't a book I knew anything about. I had never heard of it or had any intention of buying that day. That day on December 11, 2008, I was gifted this book by God. He showed me the book, took me down the aisle of books, reading or buying wasn't even on my mind. I'm guessing God knew I needed to read the book, understand the message, and get ready for my journey. What was a thought 100 miles back became a reality in my hands, all in the same day. A day that shook my world also became a day that I was gifted with a book to help me along my journey.

Life is full of gifts; we just need to keep our eyes and hearts open to search them out. The key is to **NEVER GIVE UP.**

◆ ◆ ◆

How about an uplifting exercise? Take a few minutes and write out a miracle that you have experienced—think on it, write it out, and enjoy the journey.

My miracle:

____

____

____

____

____

____

a snapshot from my journey

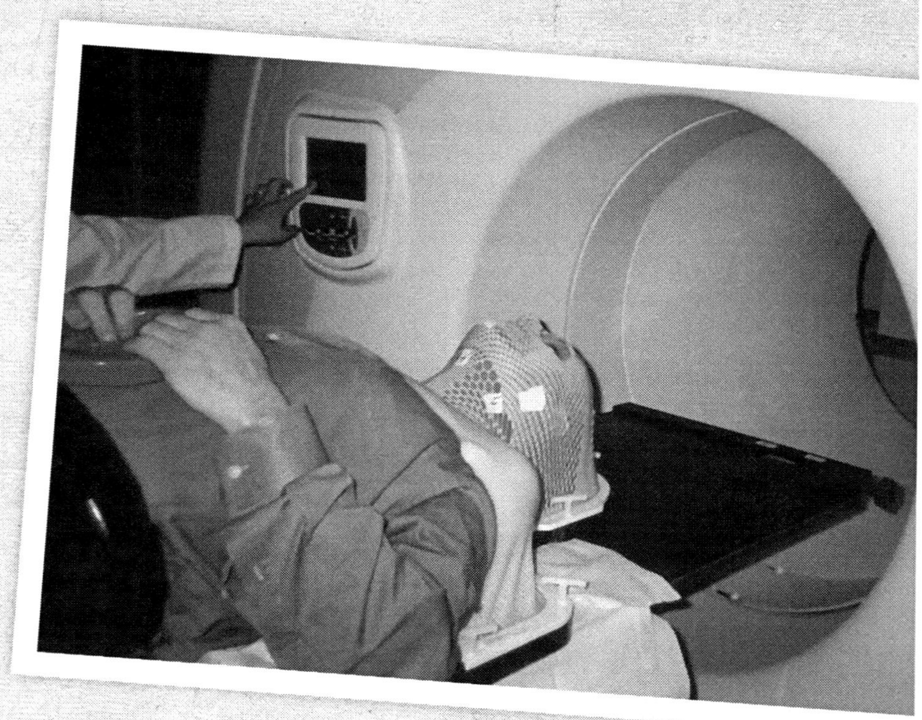

My first day of radiation treatments. This was number one of thirty, just twenty-nine to go! Even though you can't see them in this picture, I had my new tennis shoes on, purchased just before the treatments. My thinking was I would need to have a new step in my walk, and keep climbing those steps. New tennis shoes were a must!

◆ ◆ ◆

Change is okay, no matter what the change may be.
Life is about constant, exciting change.
—Larry S. Cockerel, The Cancer-Fighting Specialist

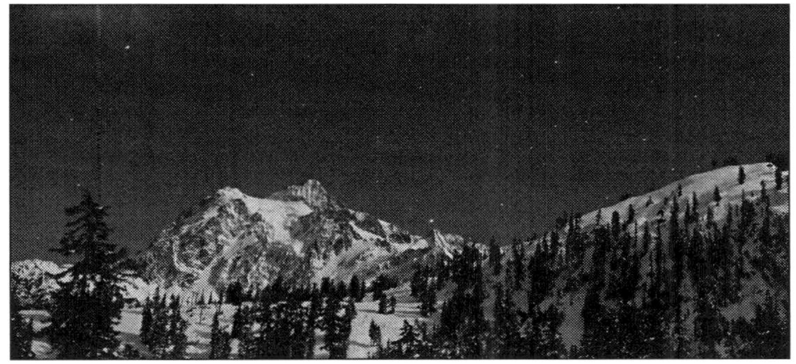

If you'll search, you will find—

change is okay

...Cancer doesn't have to define us.
Staying the course

My first day of radiation treatments went pretty fast. They got me in, checked my weight like they did at every appointment, and then had me go into the treatment room, take off my glasses, loosen my shirt, and lie down to get my mask fitted and then line everything up. I would wait for them to say "You're ready now." This stuff was scary and I'm not going to lie to you, folks. That machine was scary looking. What if the radiation hit the wrong spot or place? What if something went wrong? Everyone there made me feel very comfortable. A great team of experts, but what if? That is what was going through my mind, and then I would just shut my eyes and think and pray. I had my brand new tennis shoes on for my first treatments and I remember them saying "I see you got new tennis shoes for the occasion" and I would say "Yes, I have my mountain to climb and my race to win here."

Change was happening in my life and it was happening fast.

I believe that most people are searching for their purpose, their mission in life, their place in this world. I know that I have and I still am. I've also discovered that nothing stays the same. What you may think is your life purpose and mission can change, can improve, can offer different paths, depending on what season in life you may be in, or what's happening in your life—good or bad.

I'm a searcher, a thinker, and a believer that there is something much bigger than me and you. I believe if you search, you'll find things that may scare you, intrigue you, excite you, and change you.

Certainly, cancer isn't something we search for. It finds us, then we search for the answers and the answers will change us. Change is okay. It prepares us, molds us, and gets us excited about new things. Change can also redefine us, lift us, and prepare us for the unknown. Change is going to happen, regardless. The question is, are we in control of the change that's going to happen?

Cancer can change our thinking in either a positive or negative way. It can control our thinking very easily if we allow it to. Cancer can cause us to not want to change, and accept the negative aspects of the disease. This cancer thing is strong, deep, and deadly—not only physically but worse, mentally and psychologically. It's imperative that we stay focused on living and changing our thinking to adapt to the change that will occur.

Think about this: our world is creating and re-creating itself every second. If our perceptions shape reality, then we are creating the future every moment, and everything we think and do can determine how things play out.

I read once that the Buddhists believe that the end of all suffering is acceptance. Accept what's happening to you now. Don't run from it. You can't hide; it's as real as you are. You cannot run away from yourself. *Wherever You Go, There You Are* is a wonderful book by John Kabat-Zinn—and a great philosophy to live by.

If you'll search, you'll find the power and desire to live, to give, the purpose to keep moving forward with your treatments, the pain, and the unknown. The rewards can be greater than all the pain. I was able to keep moving forward through the 30 (six weeks) radiation treatments and chemotherapy days, despite all the changes that were happening to me and around me. I kept focused on what was important in my life, not the cancer.

Speaking about focus, the first time I went in to get fitted for my "radiation mask" was the real meaning of focus and change. It was a strange experience and a little scary if I may say. They took the time to have me lie down on the bed that moved in the tomotherapy radiation machine with my mask fitted very tightly. The team there told me that my comfort level would increase as the treatments went on. They were right; I had to stay focused on making it comfortable. There was no pain in the process itself; it was quick and easy. The picture of my mask will always take me back to the first day and the last day of radiation treatments, the beginning and

◆　◆　◆

Yes, that's me in all my colors, all my beauty! The Mask is what I call it, should have brought it home with me. I kick myself today. This could have been another trophy for my wall of fame, or not!

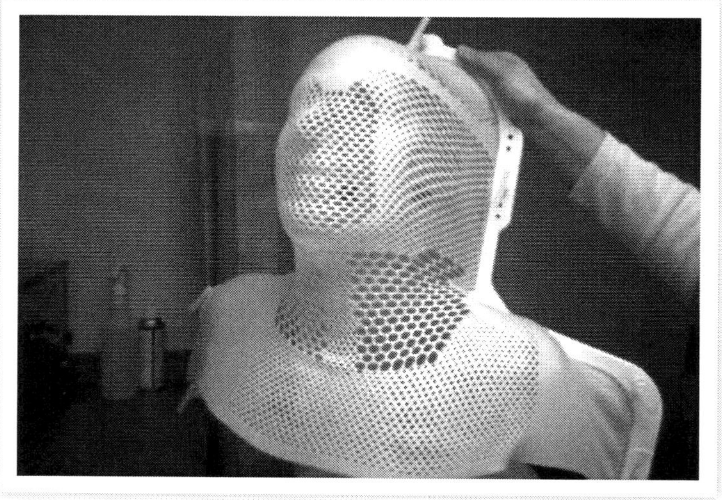

the end of my treatments. Change is okay, it has to be okay, and I had to change my thinking and dial up my courage for the battle.

This experience was all about change…

I've learned over the years that change is okay. If something's not working, change it. If my attitude isn't right, change it. If the direction I'm going isn't leading me to my highest priority goals, change it. Change is okay and it's going to happen. Change is good when it leads to positive results. Changing your thinking can change your insight and focus.

Cancer forces us to change our lifestyle. It moves us to change our habits, our attitudes, our behaviors. It can change the people around us and their attitudes, habits, and behaviors as well. It can run our lives if we allow it to.

Through our innate ability to change, adapt, and grow daily, we are in a constant state of creation. Think about the following, which I believe goes hand in hand with the reasoning that "change is okay."

Our bodies create new cells every moment. We replace the trillions of cells in our bodies every seven years. We are constantly being reborn in the flesh. That is a powerful way to say that change is okay! Each of us is changing every second of every day. Our bodies are constantly changing as we age. I've found that what matters most is the change within us, our thinking, our self-esteem, the way we look at what comes our way, the cancer and the treatments.

Every morning, we are renewed and healed. We have a brand-new day to change our world by changing our thinking about our world. No one said that life is fair. In fact, it isn't. However, what we think about, how we respond or react, how we choose to think about things, can determine how fair we make it for ourselves. Think about being reborn every day. Face the changes cancer brings head on. Face your fears, change your thinking to empower you, and keep moving.

Man has climbed the tallest mountains, walked on the moon, separated cells, discovered the power of DNA, taught the blind to read and the mute to communicate, and replaced hearts and human limbs. We have built the tallest buildings and most powerful microprocessors, computers that can store more information than we can imagine. Man has evolved for thousands of years, created and built cities, trains, planes, and automobiles. We have turned trees into paper and developed satellites that can see the world in many different views.

The medical community has discovered cures and medicines to relieve pain and help people to walk again. We have developed processes for almost everything; we are the most powerful living creatures on the planet. We humans can do almost anything a person can think about. As of today, there is no cure for most cancers, but there are more people living longer today who have been diagnosed with cancer than ever before in our history.

Treatment options available today continue to improve. Technology, with respect to laser-focused radiation and many other options, is wide open for most people. The laser-focused radiation treatments to specific areas and the different levels of chemotherapy to reduce sickness and pain, are better today than five years ago. Researchers continue to explore and find treatments that can improve the quality of life. Remember, there is something bigger than cancer: hope, and the desire to live to give. Hope, my friend, is bigger than cancer, bigger than the pain, bigger than the treatment options.

◆ ◆ ◆

My Life Formula

A famous formula in my line of work is:

E + R = O, **E**vent plus **R**esponse equals **O**utcome

I use it in both my personal and professional life to constantly remind myself that I am in charge of choosing the outcome. I also recommend it to people in my training courses to help simplify most situations. Here's how it works:

The *event* in this case is cancer. The *response* is comprised of my attitude, my faith, and my ability to change and adapt, as well as my willingness to go through the treatments. My *outcome* is then determined mentally, spiritually and physically.

Another event could be a treatment. My response: whatever I have to do, I'll pay the cost. My outcome: it's behind me today.

Give the formula a try. Practice it. My hope is that it can work for you in most of your life situations. Let the **E+R=O** formula work for you. Don't let the "event" cancer define you. Allow your "response" to be your will, your power, your motivation to lead you to your "outcome," a life to keep living and giving.

The Power Within

Here's a quote for you to think about by John C. Maxwell, from his book, *Put Your Dream to the Test:*

> *For most people, the limitations they face aren't on the outside, only on the inside.*

When you search, you will find a power within you that you may not even be aware of yet. If you allow yourself to change your thinking about the cancer and your treatments, you'll find a power to keep living.

Cancer helped me to discover and even more deeply focus on my attitude and courage. The outside factors were my treatments, the check-ups, the feeding tube, but the inside factors were my ability and desire to keep moving and not "camping out" in my cancer. I believe we all harness a deep power of faith and determination, and when faced with life's rough edges, we must unleash this power. I saw a real power of faith in our decisions and trust from Debbie when all this started. There was a lot of fear of the unknown, my health, my life, my job, our financial situation. I know this all surrounded Debbie, but she was strong, and together we climbed the mountain.

Here are some more inspiring numbers. There are over 200 billion stars in our galaxy, and we keep searching to learn more, to understand our planet and our purpose. I read once that we have over 20 billion memory cells in our brain. (Who counted them all, I wonder?) Why do we need to know this? Because of hope, the need to know more, to learn more, to give more. There is something greater than your cancer and that's you!

There Is Something Greater Than Cancer—You!

Just look at *Jerry's Kids*, the Labor Day MDA Telethon. Hope and the desire to live to give, are bigger than any cancer or illness. Hope is key to the success of our future with respect to cancer treatments. Hope can give you the edge to keep living, to keep changing and adapting to the treatments and the unknown. Living to give is why we keep getting closer to a cure.

To conquer your dreams, to keep a strong attitude, to never give up, you must be willing to change, no matter what the cost. Living overrules the pain. Love outreaches the treatments. Cancer can't take away our ability to love, to give, to listen, to hold another's hand, to go for walks. Cancer can't control our thinking, our ability to smile, or offer our smiles as a gift to another cancer traveler.

It's not our choice to get cancer. It's a disease within us. It's not you. You have your mind and heart; you can still touch and hug someone. You are a powerful living person, not the cancer. Pick up your cross and march on, run your race, climb your mountain, don't just lie down and quit. Keep living and enjoying your gift of life each day that you can. When you have one of those day's where you have no energy, or feel sick, just sit back and think good thoughts, think of your good days and those you love. That is what I did on my bad days. I slowed down and thought good thoughts. I did what I needed to do to change my thinking and get motivated to keep moving.

◆ ◆ ◆

It's Not About Cancer; It's About You

Don't limit your thinking, your ability to live. Don't allow the cancer to be greater than you. Accept your situation and attack it from all sides. You are greater than the cancer. You have the drive, desire, and passion to keep living. You have dreams to conquer, new people to meet and encourage through your journey, and you have the right to live your best life. You are God's gift to others, with a greater purpose than you can ever imagine.

a snapshot from my journey

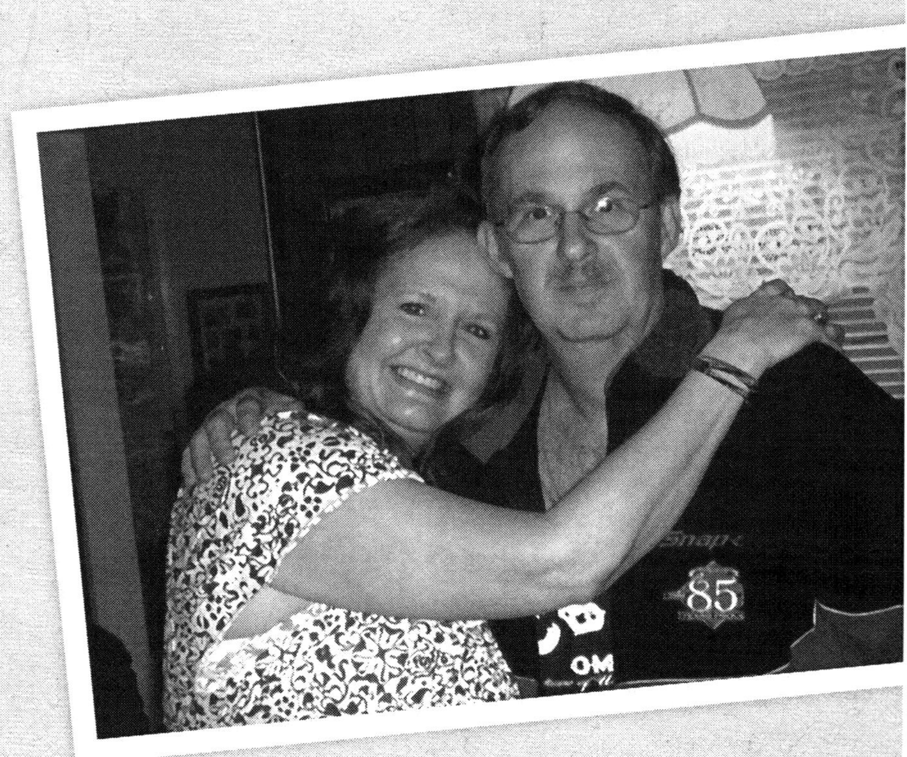

My loving sister Rene and me at my mother's home on Mother's Day, my surprise visit! The 24-hour round trip gave me many hours to reflect, not so much on what I had just gone through and the cancer, but where I needed to go and what I wanted to achieve in life.

◆ ◆ ◆

Encourage others: Mother's Day 2009, four weeks after radiation treatments, with feeding tube still in, I drove to Cabot, Arkansas to surprise my family and to prove that I could do it. I was alive!

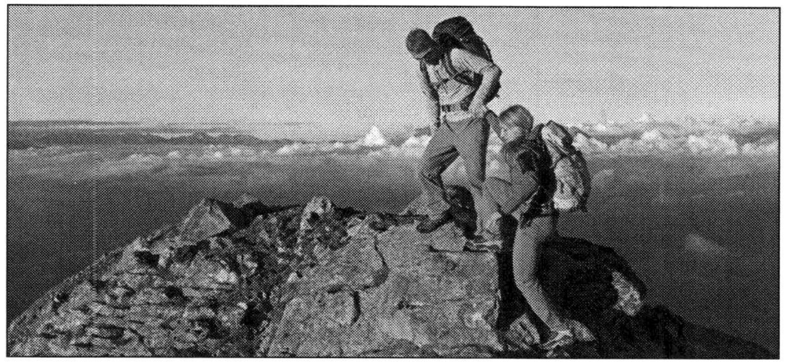

Learn to live life thoughtfully—

encourage others

*...There is something greater
than cancer—You!*

As I think of encouragement, I think back of all the little things my sister Rene did for me the days before and after my surgery and throughout my treatments. I would get cards and little text messages of encouragement, hope, and love. She never gave up on me and I didn't give up on myself. None of us really knew what to expect from the surgery and the treatments and the worst case scenario of what if cancer comes back?

The power of encouragement was a gift to me from my sister during those days. As I reflect back over the years, my sister was there many times for me. What a life partner! I would get her little notes and cards and my tears would flow. I felt loved so much even though she was over 700 miles away in Arkansas. Encouragement can come from miles away to right in front of your face to a hug from Debbie before she left for work each day. I've accepted that today I must repay the world for all the encouragement I have received over the years. I have been blessed with cancer, love, encouragement, and the ability to give back. My trip to Arkansas on Mother's Day 2009 was awesome. I hoped to encourage my family by showing them, "I'm back and on my way!"

I decided to make the trip with my medication, feeding tube, plenty of Ensure®, hope, and the self-encouragement to keep living and moving through my cancer journey.

Life is a continuous, decision-making process. Choices determine our daily successes, our journey, our relationships, and our ability to fight the cancer.

"I have cancer, but cancer doesn't have me." I completely accepted that mindset. One day, I'm going to walk away from any connection with it (cancer), I kept telling myself. Some of you might say, "Larry, that isn't realistic thinking. You're living in a fog, a state of confusion." I say, "It's my choice and my decision to think that I have cancer, but it doesn't have me and

I don't want to have anything to do with it. I choose to want to live to give, to live thoughtfully. To be able to live this way, I must learn to reject the negative and only focus on the positive outcomes," no matter what comes my way.

Cancer is a disease; we're not the disease. Cancer is a cell, not a human being. Cancer can't be seen with the human eye except though a microscope, but our loved ones, our friends, our children, are ever so visible. Cancer can't take away our spirit, our love, our memories, our hopes and dreams. Cancer can destroy our bodies, the containers in which we live, like a storm can destroy our homes, but it can't take away our thoughts and memories. Yes, cancer can take a life. But if that person has found peace, shared his or her love, and fought the good fight, the cancer didn't win.

Encouraging others can be a way of life if we choose it to be. We all know how good it feels to help someone, hug someone in need, do something special for another. I believe as humans, we are wired to want to give, help and be supportive towards others. The need to help, offer a helping hand, pick something up that another drops, open the door for a lady, is inherent in each of us. Giving is good. It's healthy, and it's inspiring and motivating.

The pure act of helping another person unselfishly is uplifting. When you know someone is in need, someone you know and care about it, there is this deep desire to help, to reach out. Life is good. It's even better than good when we can help another or encourage someone who needs encouragement.

For me, the cancer journey has created a deep need to want to help others even more than before, to make a difference.

Learning to live life thoughtfully starts at home, meaning with you. I must want to live this lifestyle, accept this mindset. To be able to achieve this, I must keep a clear mind and a laser-focused mindset of good thoughts. To live thoughtfully is to think of others first and to be kind and courteous. I believe this lifestyle can help me get better faster, and get rid of the cancer sooner. The more thoughtful I am to others, the more thoughtful I will be to myself.

Have you ever heard of the "30-Second Rule"? Within the first thirty seconds of coming into contact with someone, acknowledge the good, compliment that person, smile and say something nice and encouraging. I practice this rule, which I have dubbed "Larry's Law of Encouragement," whenever I have the opportunity. It's a great way of connecting. And when you practice it, you will feel better about yourself. An added bonus: others will want to help you more along your life journey.

Living a life of thoughtfulness toward others can only help me be kinder to myself, more appreciative of my gifts and what I have. I've been blessed to still be alive today to write to you. I have my life with Debbie and my family and friends. I see my purpose ever more strongly, to offer hope and encouragement to others. I believe that my cancer journey has opened my eyes to a new life, a more rewarding life, and a more thoughtful life.

Cancer can do many things to us. It can force us to give up or move up. Here are 15 thoughts about what cancer can do in a thoughtful way:

- Cancer can force us to feel sick or give to the sick.

- Cancer can cause us pain or help us gain a clear mindset.

- Cancer can invite us to sorrow or help us give ourselves to others.

- Cancer can take away our hope or help us hope for more.

- Cancer can cause worry and stress or teach us what not to worry about.

- Cancer can lead us to drift away from our faith or bring us closer to a faithful life.

- Cancer can cause us monetary losses or show us new riches.

- Cancer can mess up our thinking or help us focus our thoughts.

- Cancer can scare us or strengthen our weaknesses.

- Cancer may come back or be gone for good.

- Cancer may cause sickness or teach us about healthy living choices.

- Cancer can shorter our life, but it can't steal our dreams.

- ◆ Cancer can cause us to feel guilty or we can take responsibility of our body, mind, and soul.

- ◆ Cancer can confuse us or we can decide to think clearly.

- ◆ Cancer can take away, but we can live to give, thankfully, thoughtfully, and faithfully.

Yes, cancer can do lots of damage, but we can do more good by choice. Cancer is a monster in itself, but we are greater. We have minds, desires, passions, and drive. Cancer doesn't have a mind, or goals, or skills, or friends. Cancer doesn't have the ability to encourage another or offer hope. Cancer can't talk, walk, or touch. Cancer can't hug another person, or offer a smile or a warm cup of coffee. Cancer can't steal our dreams or hope unless we allow it to. Cancer can't drive us to treatments and hold our hand. Cancer can't offer us a present, or be by our side when we need someone. Cancer can't breathe. It can't hear us crying or laughing. Cancer can't take us out to dinner and be a friend. Cancer can't have a friendly conversation with us and offer us love. There are a lot of things that cancer can't do compared to what life offers you and me.

Cancer has taught me to live life more thoughtfully, more faithfully, and more thankfully. Cancer has taught me to not take my life for granted. The ability to encourage others and to offer hope has turned into a deeper passion than I could ever have imagined. This passion is good, and it came from evil. Cancer has opened my eyes to a deeper life of giving. Cancer has no mercy, but it can teach us to have mercy. What is bad and evil can teach us to love others more deeply, more considerately, and with greater passion.

Life with cancer can be good, can be rewarding, and can be shareable. Life after cancer can be lived more thankfully. No matter where you are along your cancer journey, your life can be a blessing to another, your story can help lift another person's spirit. Your daily wins can offer encouragement to another without hope. Your love for life can help others with the pain and the confusion. Take this thing called cancer and turn it around, make a U-turn in your thinking. Discover what it can make you, and then offer these gifts to others for encouragement.

Life is worth living when we are living not just for ourselves, but for others. Learn to live life thoughtfully by encouraging others daily. Discover that cancer can help you grow. Take the sour and make something sweet out of it, like taking lemons and making lemonade. Living a life of giving and sharing our experiences with those who are having tougher times is why we were created. If we are God-like, which I believe, then our mission is to take our experiences and help others along their journey. Cancer is bad, but the lessons we can learn through the cancer journey are priceless. Whether you have cancer or another life-threatening illness, you can learn through life's lessons. If we seek, and search for the honey, the sweetness of life's offerings awaits us.

Our lifestyle is our choice and what we do with this thing called cancer can either make us or break us. A thoughtful lifestyle can be so rewarding. I do my best every day to offer hope, add value, listen to understand while someone is talking, and asking myself how I can offer hope and encouragement through my life experiences. You don't have to be a writer, speaker or trainer to offer hope and encouragement. No matter what you do in life, you have something to offer and give to others. No matter how much you give today, there is always tomorrow and more experiences to share.

Learning to live thoughtfully is really quite simple. It takes a positive attitude, an unselfish outlook, a "givers-gain" mindset, and the willingness to help others first before seeking our own rewards. I've found that the more that I can do for others, the better I feel, and the better I feel, the stronger I am physically. Could it be that the better we think and feel, the better we can fight the good fight for life?

Living thoughtfully is easy. Simply be thoughtful to the first person you come into contact with daily. First and foremost, be thoughtful and kind to yourself. Think to yourself, "What can I say, what can I do, to be thoughtful, to be courteous?" Then act, take the first step. Be the person you want to be. Think like a person who cares about others. Big tip: This is part of the recovery process. I believe the more we can think good thoughts towards others and do for others, the more we will gain new strength to fight the cancer.

Throughout this journey with cancer, I have asked myself many questions, like: How have I lived this gift of life that

I've been given? How have I made a difference? Whom have I impacted?

The thought of cancer, chemotherapy, radiation treatments, and the possibility of the cancer coming back even worse than the first time, is terrifying. I also catch myself asking, "How long do I have? Am I healthy? What can I do differently with the blessed time that I'm gifted with?

I sit and wonder at times, "Is it back? Is it building itself to attack again? Have I controlled the monster?" I would be willing to bet that these questions are floating around in your mind, too. Only time will tell. I know that no matter what, I will never give up. I'll climb the mountain one step at a time. I'll keep dreaming of a better life and I'll manage my attitude towards the journey to stay focused to my course and my vision for a good life. If I'm going to think, I might as well think big, right?

◆ ◆ ◆

My Daily Success Is Determined By The Seeds I Sow, Not The Harvest I Reap

The ability to encourage another is a gift, an ability that lies deep within us. If we all lived according to this philosophy, the world might experience fewer wars, diseases, hurt, crime, and negative environments. Think about choosing to live according to the Golden Rule: *do unto others as you would have done unto you.* The philosophies we live by are our choice. Our mindset and our positive attitude are our choices.

To be "human givers," we must learn to encourage ourselves to keep living and enjoying life, to be able to offer encouragement to others. To dream of a life full of love, friends, family, and a healthy lifespan, we must encourage our faith, our thankful thinking, and our thoughtfulness towards ourselves, the cancer, and life.

If I'm going to live in the now and enjoy the day, I might as well think this way every day that I'm blessed with. If God is going to gift me with another year, or five years, or ten, I might as well do something big with that gift, right? I've chosen to conquer my dreams and think good thoughts with a positive and enthusiastic attitude about life. I'm accepting the fact that change is okay and my mission is to encourage as many people as I can along my journey. These are my daily choices. What are yours?

Take a good look at yourself. What do you see? What do you want to see? Can you see a person who cares about himself or herself so much that he or she will do anything to get better, pay the cost of treatments, and live to give another day? Do you see a person who cares about others so much that it encourages you to keep living, just to be able to give again to those that you love and need you?

You can only give what you have. In life, you can learn to give, you can enhance your strengths, your abilities; you can grow and develop your passions. You can climb the tallest mountains; you can fight the good fight for life. The best thing is you don't have to fight the cancer alone. There are many others who want to connect and encourage, and you have friends and family. You also have God to help you along your journey.

How do we learn to encourage others? First, we must learn to encourage ourselves. The cancer journey has taught me much about enjoying life and living life to my fullest potential, and my fullest potential includes others, just as your life does. Cancer has taught me to keep fighting, keep growing, and to keep enjoying life through others. Cancer has taught me that life is short and precious, fragile and simple. Cancer has taught me that living to give is part of the healing process, a key piece to my self-encouragement and growth.

Encourage others. Reach out and find another cancer patient and ask what you can do to offer hope, a smile, and a little laughter. Let the other person know that you've hit the wall, too, that you're still climbing your mountain, and you are still living to give. Find a friend to talk with, to share your story, your good days, and your low days. Find a buddy who understands your journey, your pain, and your fears. Find a new friend who has traveled where you are headed, has been through the treatments you are facing. Find a friend you can cry with, you can laugh with, someone who understands.

Search for another to encourage. Feel the good feeling of love, the warm feeling of giving. Share your story of recovery, your fear of treatments. Talk about the journey, don't hide from it. Don't be afraid. Face the giant, win the battle, live to give one step at a time, one day at a time.

When it comes to encouraging others, it's also about how others encouraged me. From my medical team at each meeting, to Debbie just coming home to me, my family being there for me on my surgery day to my little "Cancer-Fighting Team" at home (Debbie + the cats). Then there are those who can't be there for you in a physical state, like Steve Schultz who kept calling me to see if I needed a ride to treatments, which would have been a six-hour day for him. And then my sister Rene, who sent me texts daily, cards, and Bible verses to lift my spirits. There were so many. I believe that I could write a small book of inspiration just from all the love and encouragement that came my way during this trying period in my life.

Something very special came to me in the mail from my oldest niece, Serena. It came on one of those hard days, and lifted my soul, spirit and brought tears to my eyes, just when I needed it, during the weeks after treatments when life was really hard. The gift was simple, creative, homemade, and one of a kind! The best kind of gift you can get, not store-bought, but made with love and by the hands of one of my sweet little nieces.

Encouragement can come in many different ways, a hug, a card, phone call, special visit, or just someone sitting with you in your chemotherapy room as support.

Let me get back to the special gift that arrived on a day when I really needed a lift, some extra love and it came in a 9 x 11 envelope and now will stay in my office with all my things that hang from the walls and decorate the desk area.

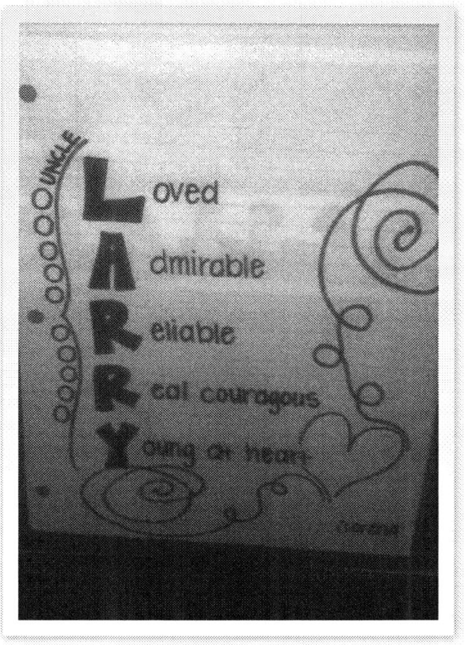

You know what I mean: all the good stuff in life, my museum. My special "LARRY" meaning of life! What a gift of encouragement. It's so easy to lift another, offer encouragement, and show our love. Why do we not do it more often, is the question? I love my family and I know they love me and that is about that best form of encouragement to never give up and keep living and enjoying my gift of life. Serena, I thank you and I love you!

Live your life thoughtfully, faithfully, and thankfully each day. Be a blessing to another. Lift a friend's spirits. Visit the lonely. Love your spouse and kids more intensely and more deeply than ever before. Don't stop living and giving, conquering your dreams, climbing your highest mountain. Don't let the cancer be all about the cancer; make it be all about you. Make the choices that will lead you to a healthy and positive attitude about where you are and where you're going. It is what it is, right? Decide to make healthy choices.

Everybody needs someone. Everyone wants to be heard and understood. Everybody wants to be someone. Today is your time, your time to encourage another, be human, be friendly, be approachable, and reach out and touch someone. No matter where you are along your journey in life, there is always someone who needs more, who needs encouragement, hope, and to know that there can be a good life with and after cancer.

Today is your day. Live to give and enjoy this gift of life that you have been blessed with. Go out and be a blessing to someone else. If it's true that one out of three people we encounter may have some form of cancer, you're not far away from your next opportunity to be a blessing. Feel the good feeling of giving and enjoy it. I hope that my words of encouragement have inspired you to go out and inspire someone you know who needs it. We are never alone; we just need to connect, share, inspire, smile, listen, and love. Just like God waits for us, others are waiting for our encouragement, our love and our courage. We do not walk this world alone, unless we choose to.

It Is What It Is!

Debbie gifted me with a wooden sign to hang over our fireplace that says; *It Is What It Is*! I love that saying. We can't wave off the cancer; once it's alive, it is what it is. It is what it is... when something happens that you have no control over—an accident, a bad relationship, the weather, or cancer... it is what it is!

There have been many "it is what it is" occurrences in my life, from career changes, relationships, bad financial decisions, good calls, and bad calls. I'd be willing to bet that you have used this statement or read it or even lived it as I have. When the doctor says you have cancer, it is what it is. "Now what" becomes the question? This is what we talked about in a previous chapter: the "event," then the "response," then the 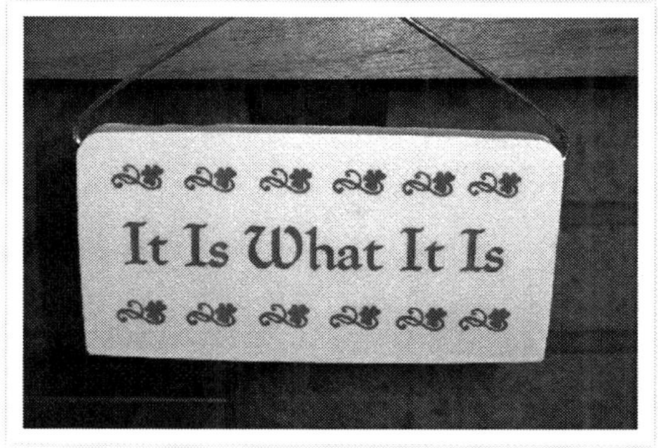

"outcome," the action or attitude to deal with the situation.

Yes, "It Is What It Is" still hangs over the fireplace. It's a good place for it. I see it often!

◆ ◆ ◆

Living Without Regrets
Don't Let The Regrets Of Yesterday Destroy The Hopes Of Tomorrow

The regrets of yesterday can be a burden on our future. The effects of what cancer can do to a good person can be earth-shattering. The regrets of yesterday can lead us down the wrong path. The key is living in the now, dealing with the day, especially when dealing with cancer and your treatments.

Don't live your life regretting what you should have done or could have done. Don't live your life today thinking, "What if I would have only done that, or this?" We can so easily fall into that trap of thinking, "What if I would have eaten better, not smoked all those years, exercised more …

Maybe if I would have... maybe the cancer would have never taken over my life."

I plead with my readers not to live a "guilt-based" life. Cancer isn't something you chose or wanted; it's just what it is, cancer. Please don't think guilty thoughts about what you should have or shouldn't have done, doesn't matter now. What matters is your positive attitude about where you want to go and your wellness.

Please don't live your life wishing for a different past, a better yesterday. I've come to accept that after 51 years, I can't do anything to change the past. Nothing. All I can do today is live my best life. There is a whole boatload of stuff I wish I wouldn't have done, shouldn't have done, but they're in the past. All that thinking will not help me fight the good fight for life against cancer. I can worry myself to death or I can grow and go. I can learn to march forward, eyes focused straight ahead, seeking a better tomorrow, and a more rewarding life with or without cancer. My hope for a better tomorrow is key to my recovery, my fight against cancer, my ability to encourage others.

Here's another very important lesson I've learned from all this cancer stuff: tomorrow awaits me, but today is my walk, my journey. Yesterday is gone, can't be changed, can be looked upon as a lesson to offer me hope and encouragement for a better day. Yesterday's regrets are just what they are: yesterday, a day that is gone from the calendar, the past. Yesterday's over, done with, no more "if only," "wish I would have's..."

When there is hope for the future, there is power to make change happen, to get better, to be stronger and healthier, to be happier—today. When tomorrow comes, it will come with a swift and quick trip. Only so many minutes and hours to live our best life. Only so many people to see and to encourage and offer hope. Tomorrow comes and it will go. How will you live tomorrow when it comes? Will you live in the present, the future, or in the past? I encourage you to live in the present— because it is truly a present. Maybe there's no bow, no wrapping paper, and no cake and ice cream, but each day is truly a present, a gift.

I've learned to love life and never give up. I've also learned to not live in the past, but to grow from my past experiences. I would not have changed a thing, a decision that was made over the past year regarding my therapy, knowing what I know today. I have no regrets about yesterday, only praises. I have no regrets about my journey with cancer, couldn't have changed it if I wanted to. It was alive and present. It was my time to step up and not give up or give in but fight to win my battle, just as David fought his battle with Goliath.

My hope for tomorrow was greater than the fear that stood in front of me. My hope and dreams outweighed the cancer. My love for life and Debbie and my family was greater than the cancer. My God was bigger than the cancer and my faith was stronger. I chose to never give up, to keep a solid, positive attitude, and to accept the cards I had been dealt. My hope for a better tomorrow was and is my inspiration.

What is your inspiration? What dreams will keep you moving through your cancer? What are you willing to pay and do? Please don't settle in your past or yesterday's treatments. Instead, look forward, reach for tomorrow, live to grow and give. Tomorrow is much more exciting than yesterday. I don't care how wonderful yesterday was—tomorrow is your future, your opportunity to live and enjoy your gift of life. Make it a gift by giving yourself to others; share your story, your courage, and your faith.

◆　◆　◆

Taking Control Of The Future

I made the decision that the feeding tube was coming out two weeks before its scheduled removal date. I chose to step up and move forward. I contacted the hospital and asked them to schedule a time to remove my feeding tube. It was time to force myself to get back to a "normal" state of mind and eat regular food. It was time to let go of yesterday and reach for tomorrow. It was time to let go of that part of treatment and get well faster. On that day, it only took a few minutes to remove the tube, and I was free. My tomorrow was looking better every second, every minute. I was on the road to recovery. This was my choice of thinking. Remember, it's a choice on how we choose to think.

Our Thinking Determines Our Attitudes

Get out of your bed, remove the feeding tube a week earlier if you're able to, drive yourself to your treatments, do what your medical team recommends, don't ever give up on yourself. It's your life, it's your time; don't let cancer stand in the way. Turn it into a stepping stone for a better tomorrow, a tomorrow full of hope and excitement. Give it all you've got. I understand that these recommendations won't work for everyone, but I encourage you to expand your thinking, take the risk, and step up to your cancer the best you can and face your giant head on.

If I had yesterday to live over again, what would I do differently? I would live more thoughtfully, thankfully, and faithfully. I would design my life around giving, a life of joy, and loving my family even more deeply than the day before. If I had yesterday to live again, I would take my treatments, I would feed myself through the tube, and I would get up in the morning with hope for a better day. I would live to give and encourage. If I had yesterday to live again, I would live it with no regrets, only hope for a better tomorrow.

If you had yesterday to live again, what would you do differently? Would you live for the day and hope for a better tomorrow? How would you handle the gift of another day? Live it with no regrets, no second questioning your actions, no "if only," no "should have's." Live in the present and enjoy the present. The gift of life is yours to live, to give, to inspire, to encourage and to love. I hope your mission will include conquering your dreams, having a great attitude about life, never giving up, changing, and encouraging yourself and others.

a snapshot from my journey

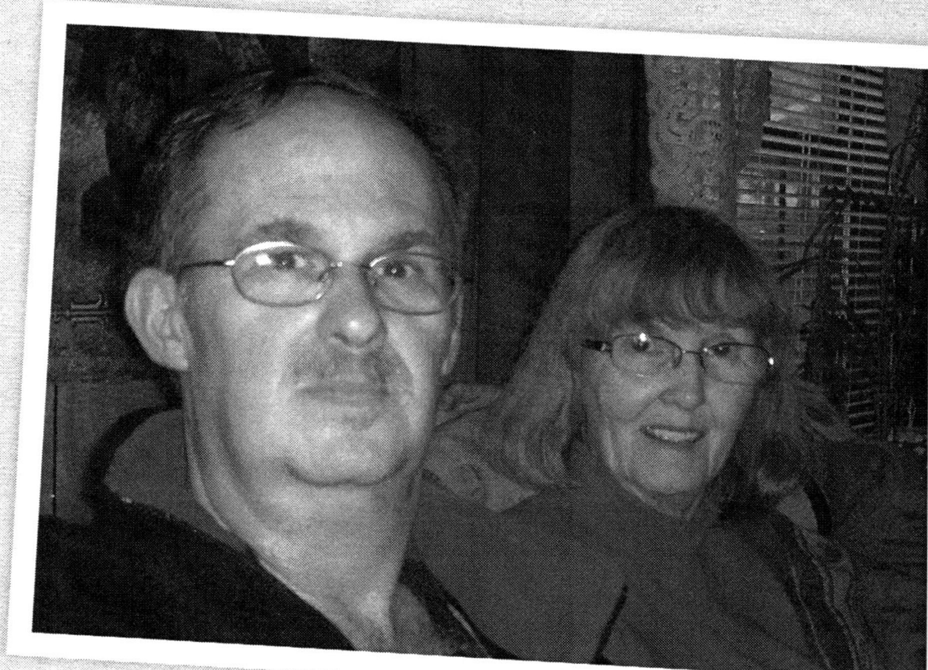

My exciting 24-hour round trip to Cabot, Arkansas, 4 weeks after treatments, with the feeding tube in. I couldn't eat most things, had lost 40-plus pounds, was tired, but still strong in will. The trip helped me use the time to reflect and grow so that I could keep going!

◆　◆　◆

"Be happy with what you've got!" My mother JoAnne and me on Mother's Day, 2009. The ability to reflect on where I've been helps me to get to where I want to go.

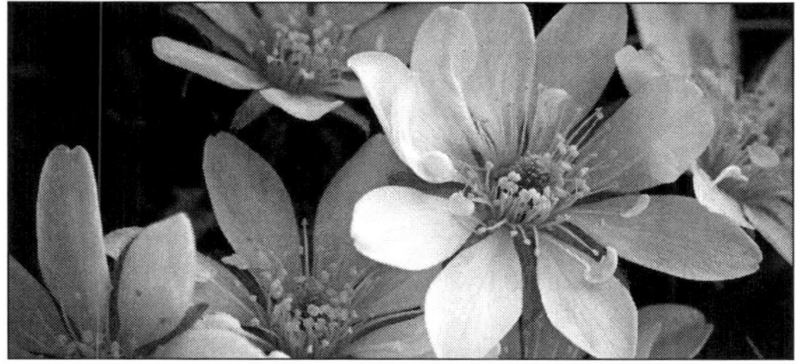

Be happy with what you've got—

reflect
and grow

...Don't let the regrets of yesterday destroy the hopes of tomorrow

Mother's Day 2009 was what we call a "tipping point." That trip did a few things: First was a big surprise for my mother (Joanne) and my family, second was providing me with a time to reflect and grow from my experience and third, to learn how good a food buffet was for me. The trip helped to motivate my recovery and share my love with my family. The time was short but powerful.

I showed up at my mother's home ready to surprise them and guess what? No one was home! I waited for almost an hour and half before they showed up, made some phone calls to other family members, but no answers. Tired and ready to get out of the car, I waited. When finally they showed up, I went to the front door, and I believe I did a good job of gifting a mother with one of the best gifts she could get: her son home on Mother's Day, six weeks after cancer treatments with a feeding tube hanging out of my stomach!

This is what it's all about: being happy with what you've got. Be happy with where you're at in life. Be happy with those you love and who love you. Be happy about your recovery, your remission, your therapy, your strength. Be happy with what you have while you reach for more: more to give and to live.

Throughout my cancer journey, I learned more and more about what life is about. It's not about getting, but giving; it's not about taking, but sharing. Life is about being happy with where I'm at, with what I have, and with whom I'm blessed having in my life. I've also learned that time is more important than money; I can always get more money, but I can't get any more time.

Sure, there was a time in my life where "things" were most important: cars, bikes, motorcycles, clothes, and dinners out, vacations I couldn't afford. Now, being happy with *where* I'm at in life is much more important than what I *have* in life.

What makes you happy today? Are you happy with what you have? Are you happy with how you're dealing with your treatments? I don't expect for you to be happy about having cancer, but it's okay to be happy you're alive and that there is hope. Happiness is a feeling, an emotional decision, just like the feelings of being angry, fearful, mad and sad. It's all a choice.

Being happy with what you've got can inspire you to learn more so that you can give more. We can't give what we do not have. We can share our stories and experiences, we can help others to be happy, but we can't *make* them happy. For instance, I can't make you happy, mad, sad or glad—I can invite you to feel feelings, but I can't make you feel any particular way.

We use the phrases, "You made me sad," or "You made me happy," or "You make me feel good." None of those are really true. No one else can make us feel one way or another—feelings and emotions are an inside job. We can't make anyone other than ourselves feel a particular emotion. Of course, we can encourage, inspire, invite, and ignite an environment of good feelings, but we can't make anyone *feel.*

Cancer cannot make me feel bad, or sad, or even glad. Cancer cannot make me feel any emotions. The thoughts of cancer can invite us to make the choices to feel a certain way. It cannot control our emotions, unless we allow it to, through our choices to feel a certain way because of the cancer, or treatments. Chemo can make us sick, tired, weak, ill, uncomfortable, and even nauseous. It can change our physical beings but not our emotional mindset, unless we choose. Our choices on how we think and feel can determine our success with treatment.

Was I to be happy with what I got—cancer? No. Was I going to beat myself up about it? No. Instead, I told myself, "I'm going to put all my training, motivational stuff, personal development, and my strengths to help me through this thing." And they did!

Be happy with what you've got. Yes, even cancer. If you got it, it is what it is. No turning back, no turning off the light switch, no changing yesterday. It is what it is. But there is something that we can do to help us along our journey of recovery and wellness—and that is to reflect and grow.

As I reflect back over the past two years, I learned much about myself, Debbie, our life together, our abilities to work together, to achieve, and to overcome obstacles. I've been able to understand myself better, my capabilities, my strength zones, my weaknesses, and my faith. The journey has taught me so many more things than just enduring the pain, the treatments, and the surgery. My experience has taken me to a new level of respect for life in general and my own life. My cancer has taught me that life is scary, and that I can be totally out of control of my own life. It has taught me that I can give my life over to the hands of others with trust. Without the trust in my medical team, I believe the road would have been much harder to travel. Cancer taught me that I must trust things that I may not be up on, people I don't know and the medical process that can scare the you-know-what out of you!

This piece of the story—the journey back to wellness—is important to me, because the cancer can come and it can reside, but it can't take my hope, dreams, or desires. The cancer can't keep me from looking forward and reflecting back. It can't keep me from growing and stretching myself to new levels. It's not about the cancer, it's all about me! That's my story and I'm sticking to it.

I have cancer…I had cancer…I had to have cancer treatments…I went through cancer treatments…I'm a cancer victim… I overcame cancer…I had cancer but cancer didn't have me. Now as I write to you in 2011 a two-year cancer survivor. I made a choice not to stay in my cancer state of mind; I made a choice to keep moving through my treatments, thinking only of my recovery.

Our thoughts, our words, and our attitudes can determine our success with our treatments and journey with cancer. Our thoughts and words can determine many different things in our life: our relationships, careers, success, health, state of mind. How we think and the words we speak can be forms of treatment, and I believe they are just as important as the treatments and medication.

Reflecting back, my mission was to keep my thinking clear and positive, my attitude in check, and my words focused on "I'm getting better, it's almost done with, and my battle is close to being won. Victory awaits me!"

All along my journey with cancer, I had many conversations and pep talks with the person in the mirror, and will continue to have positive and laser-focused conversations with myself about my well-being. I've found that I can't fool the guy in the mirror. While I was going through treatments, I would look at myself and think, "Man, I've got to gain weight … I've got to force myself to eat…Add more protein drink through that feeding tube. Whatever it takes, never give up, right?"

Looking back, my words were my stepping stones. What I told myself, how I communicated, and shared the experiences with Debbie, helped me stay focused on my true mission. I was able to beat it, get it over with, and start living my "normal" life again as fast as I could. Today, reflecting back, thinking where I was and where I am today, was truly about the passion to live, to enjoy my life and all that awaits me. I've grown more over the past year than in the past fifty.

"Reflect and grow, live and love, encourage and inspire, get well and stay well," has become my mantra, the words I live by now.

I invite you to reflect back. Revisit your past, but don't camp out there. Don't rent a room in the past. Don't move back there. Go back and measure your growth, where you were, and where you are today. In my sales and leadership training, I call these different places the "as-is state" and the "should-be state" or even the "could-be state." Where do I want to be and how am I going to get there?

What is it you do to lift yourself? What are you doing with your past experiences? Are you learning and growing? Can you describe to someone what cancer has given you, rather than taken from you?

Cancer has given me many things, just as it has taken away from me. I choose to think about the things it has given to me. That way, I have something to give. I'm asking you to expand your thinking. Don't live in the negative aspects of cancer; do something good with your journey.

It is okay to let yourself go back. Reflecting on your past experiences and growing from them are much different than living in the past. Enjoy your gift of life each day, taking each step that is required to help you get where you need to go.

What cancer taught me was to not camp out in negative experiences, to keep moving and doing whatever it is I have to do to keep enjoying my gift of life. Thinking back to our vacation in the Rockies in October 2007, I knew something wasn't right. You just know your body. I've learned it communicates with me! Those sunny, awesome, warm fall days in Colorado were the beginning of my understanding that life is not in my control. Sure, I can eat right, exercise, think good thoughts, but that little lump on my neck turned out to be one of the most deadly diseases—cancer!

Today, I write to you as a two-year cancer survivor. In 2011, I am celebrating my life and doing my best to live a good life. I also accept and acknowledge the fact anything can happen, and something will happen in my future that will not be my choice. But I must live in the present, plan for my future, reflect on my past experience and grow, and never give up on living my best life now. As I reflect on my experience with cancer, I share with you to offer hope and encouragement and want you to fight your cancer, never give-up and remember it's not about the cancer, it's about you and your life.

Blueberry Muffins

Prior to my exciting experience with this ugly thing called cancer, I would visit my favorite local coffee house, The Cedarburg Coffee Roastery. Weekend mornings, I enjoyed my trip down to the Roastery, a nice cup of java, reading, thinking, creating, and savoring their homemade treats, especially the blueberry muffins!

Yes, big fresh blueberry muffins! I would get one for myself and then pick out something special for Debbie. Then I'd head home and we would enjoy our treats together. Then **BAM!** The cancer, surgery, radiation treatments and no eating and enjoying my blueberry muffins for months. No energy and no real desire to go, no enthusiasm and the worst part, it was too hard to eat.

Weeks after treatments ended, I was able to get back to my favorite little coffee house to have a little coffee, read, and think for a spell. But I sure missed my blueberry muffins. I remember telling Tammie, the owner, about my journey and how I missed her blueberry muffins; they were like carrots dangling out for me to reach. I couldn't wait, and Tammie said, "When you're ready, they will be ready," and yes, they were. It was so good to eat and enjoy those awesome blueberry muffins again.

Sometimes it's really the little things in life that are the most important: a good cup of coffee and your favorite treat. There's nothing better after a run with radiation and chemotherapy treatments! Today, I visit my little coffee shop as often as I can. Reflect, relax, and you can bet I get a treat for Debbie and a blueberry muffin for me to go, for us to enjoy together. It's the simple, little things that help us enjoy our gift of life.

I am truly too blessed to be stressed!

Enjoy your journey!

sour cream blueberry muffins

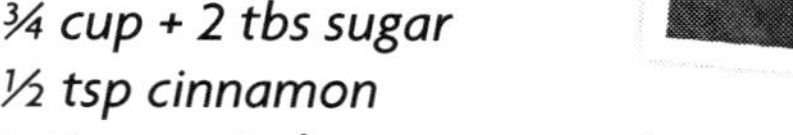

Makes 12 large muffins!

2 ¾ cups all-purpose flour
¼ cup cake flour
¾ tbs baking powder
1 tsp baking soda
1 tsp salt
¾ cup + 2 tbs sugar
½ tsp cinnamon
1 ¾ cup + 2 tbs sour cream (room temperature)
2 eggs (room temperature)
1 tbs vanilla extract
¼ pound (1 stick) butter, melted
2 ½ cups fresh blueberries
½ cup sugar
½ teaspoon cinnamon

Sift dry ingredients into a bowl and add blueberries. Mix well, careful not to crush berries. In a separate bowl, whisk together sour cream, melted butter, eggs, and vanilla until smooth. Add sour cream mixture to dry ingredients and fold together until just combined. Do not over-mix. Scoop into lined muffin tin pan and evenly sprinkle with the remaining sugar and cinnamon. Bake at 350°F for 25 to 30 minutes. (Until a toothpick comes clean out of center of muffins.)

◆　◆　◆

This is truly a gift, a secret recipe for the wonderful blueberry muffins! I see my book as a secret recipe for courage, change, and human potential. It's all about living, giving, and enjoying your gift of life with others; now enjoy a wonderful blueberry muffin together! Many thanks to my favorite little coffee house, The Cedarburg Coffee Roastery.

epilogue

As I complete this book, my story on how cancer has enhanced my life and helped me change my vision and mission, it is now 2011, two years past my surgery and treatment process. I am a two-year survivor! I'm on my way, baby!

Cancer has truly become one of my mentors. A mentor is meant to teach you so that you can teach others what you have learned. Two years have passed now since the beginning of my cancer recovery journey on January 27, 2009, my surgery day. Yes, I'm feeling good and doing better, and can't wait to get some feedback from what my story and book about what cancer has taught me has done for you.

I'll call this the final chapter, today and tomorrow. Today, I live my life as a true gift, a blessing. I do my best to aggressively live my life to its fullest potential. My hope is that this book has helped you discover that you can enjoy life by incorporating the six reasons into your personal and professional life, every moment of every day. The cancer specialist would say I'm in remission, not cured. I don't think I'll ever be completely cured; I've been kind of crazy all my life.

Today, Debbie and I live our lives daily with our two "kids," PeeWee and Peanut. We work together on conquering our dreams, with a positive attitude, never giving up on the things we want out of life for each other. Accepting that changes are going to happen, we encourage others to enjoy their gift of life. We reflect on the good times and grow together and individually live to give as much as we can in life.

My vision has changed since my cancer journey and my mission has been updated to offer hope and encouragement to everyone I meet. My vision is to enjoy life and help others enjoy their lives by adding value through my experiences.

Life is truly a blessing and a gift that is meant to be shared and lived for others. I've found that if I tried to live my life for myself alone, it would end up being a very lonely, boring life. I hope through this book and my public presentations that I can add value to others and offer hope and encouragement.

Here are a few quotes that truly inspire me:

Jim Rohn shared: *"We all have two choices. We can make a living, or design a life."*

I know that I don't want to just make a living; I truly want to design my life serving others.

John C. Maxwell offers this powerful quote about living life NOW: *"At the end, people will pick your life in one sentence. You pick it now!"*

I want to live my life the way I want to be remembered, my legacy. I want to be a man who lived his life to help others enjoy their lives no matter what challenges they may encounter.

I want to live my life bigger on the inside than on the outside. When I live my life bigger on the inside from the heart, from my passion and love for life, then my outside will never be questioned.

I hope that my book will help you enjoy your journey. And by mastering the six reasons to keep living and enjoying your gift of life, you will truly live your life to your fullest potential. Whoever thought that cancer would be one of my mentors in life?

Keep the faith, never give up, thank God daily, encourage others, look for the good and inspire someone today—that's all I ask of you. Debbie and I thank you for investing in this book; our mission is to lift another person to a higher level of well-being and encourage hope with our book and story. So who do you know who may enjoy this gift?

As you climb your mountains in life, when you get to the summit, you can look out and see the beauty of life. No matter how tough the climb and the struggle, there is beauty in the journey. I wish you the best. Be sure to enjoy the journey with those you love and sometimes even in our darkest days, we are the ones who may need to reach out our hand to help pull others up the mountain with us!

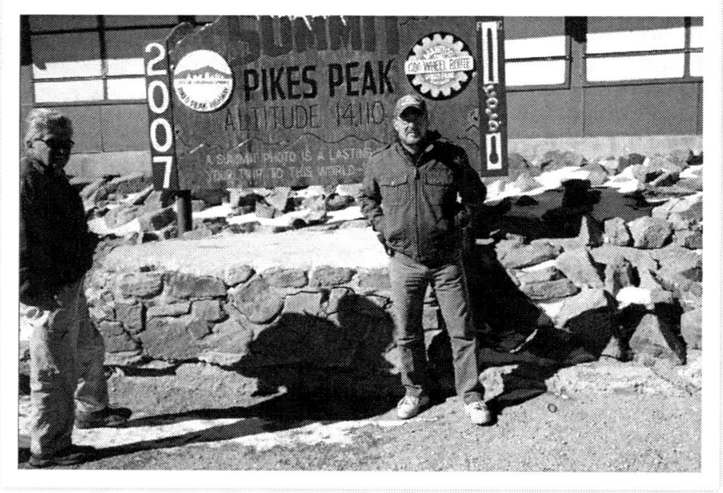

◆　◆　◆

Our vacation in the Rockies, the week of October 12, 2007, was when I first noticed this thing growing in my neck, this thing called cancer. We never gave up, we kept the right attitude, we knew change was going to happen and today we are conquering our dreams, encouraging others, and reflecting only on the good. Safe travels. Please remember happiness and success are not found in the destination but in the journey, the gift of life. Our next trip to the Rockies isn't that far away. Debbie and I can't wait!

the check-up session

In the early weeks of my radiation treatments, after each treatment I would meet with my Oncology Coordinator, Peggy W., and at least every other day, with my radiologist, Paul H. and one of his assistants. They would ask me the key question about where I rated my pain level. Early on, it was never a problem until about week four of treatments when the pain level chart made sense to me. I enjoyed the check-ups, as they allowed me to ask questions and keep myself in check. And the oncology team always offered encouragement.

This is my check-up session for you. It's time to recap the journey and offer additional hope and encouragement.

If you're reading this little book, you are still alive. Time is still your friend. You can still have hope, dreams, and others who may be counting on you, holding your hand, feeding you, bathing you, walking with you, and praying with you. Encouraging you on with your battle, walking with you, listening to you and helping you get through your battle. Your "Cancer-Fighting Team"!

Debbie was great, doing all the research on cancer, the treatments, the feeding tube, the medication—everything! She would read all the information we would get from the clinic, and mostly, just be my friend and nurturing partner each day. We all need a "Cancer-Fighting Team"— folks at the hospital or clinic, and especially the folks at home.

"I'm too blessed to be stressed." I love this quote—Think about all the blessings in your life.

I created the acronym **C.A.N.C.E.R.** for a purpose: to encourage and offer hope. I want to help others who have been touched with cancer or any other life-changing opportunity to enjoy their life and keep living and giving, and hoping for a better future. Life is truly a gift; it's what we do with that gift that makes all the difference in who we are and our purpose in life.

◆　◆　◆

Here's your follow-up visit:

Conquer Your Dreams—
The Meaning Of Life; The Journey

I believe the meaning of life is the journey: the good, the bad and the ugly. The journey offers us many opportunities. It's what we do with what comes our way that will make the difference. The journey is full of life's gifts. It's all in the gifts. Discover your gifts and give them to others and they will gift you back many times over. Conquer your dreams and enjoy your life.

The big "C" is all about conquering your dreams. That doesn't mean hoping for a dream to come true, but taking it and making it happen. Your dreams are yours. Nothing can take them away—no cancer, no illness. They will always be with you. You can learn to live them physically, as well as mentally, emotionally, and spiritually. Your dreams are yours and damn it, go for them! Don't hold back. Live your life to your fullest potential. Share it with those you love and who love you. It's your time, today is yours, tomorrow awaits you. Time is your friend.

See your dream, feel your dream, and live your dream.

Speaking of "dreams," I just finished reading an excellent book on dreams for the second time. I highly recommend you invest in this one: *Put Your Dreams to the Test: 10 Questions to Help You See It and Seize It*, by John C. Maxwell. That book has taken me to an even newer level of thinking about and conquering my dreams.

Attitude Is Everything

The "A" is all about attitude. Our "I can do this" attitude, our "I will get well" attitude, our "I'm on the right track" attitude, "I'm closer than I think" attitude, "It's not going to win" attitude, and "I'm a cancer fighter" attitude.

My words to myself along the journey with cancer were: "I'm going to live my victorious life aggressively." My positive attitude can't make everything come true, nor can it make everything better, but it's better than a negative attitude. It will take me more places than a negative outlook. My thinking at critical stages in my cancer treatments and therapy were vital to my recovery.

Cancer kills. There is no question or argument to that statement. However, there are other things that kill and are 100% under our control: our thoughts, our words, and how we choose to react or respond to the cancer. We are able to think ourselves to death. Our tongues can be just as evil as the cancer. Our words can push us over the edge; they can destroy our relationships, and our self-value. We must take control. Victory over cancer is our mission.

The words and thoughts you use can be poison or words of victory. Is attitude everything to you? Do you think a positive attitude can help you or hurt you? Do you think a positive attitude regarding your treatments and or therapy can help you get through?

It can and it will. How do we make a difference in life? Through our decisions—and our decisions are driven by our attitudes. How we think about what happens to us determines how we either react or respond. I've found that through my chemotherapy and radiation treatments, my attitude was my best friend. And I believe we need a lot of "best friends"—like attitude, perspective, desire, enthusiasm, will, and faith. It's all about choices. The choices we make, make or break us at the end of the day.

Life after treatments, our attitude toward our treatments, and our attitude about our future are all keys to our recovery and rebuilding our mind, body, and soul. We get to experience it all while traveling through this thing called cancer. It can help us to become stronger in our faith, our thankfulness for life, and pursuing our passion in life.

Battling the odds at all cost, attitude is everything. Our lives are too precious, and our attitude needs to be good, positive, and focused. Keeping the faith, having a good attitude about ourselves, focusing on the present and the future are the steps to victory.

What appears to be big, gets even bigger. We can grow from any situation, even cancer. We can see the mountain as an opportunity or a task too difficult to climb; it's our choice.

We all have mountains to climb. I encourage you to never give up, keep climbing, keep growing, keep learning, keep living and giving. The mountain can be your victory. You can stand tall and look out at all of your accomplishments. You can help others climb and you can reach down and pull others to the top with you. Victory is a choice.

Never Give Up

The "N" means never give up. We can take the cancer and make it a reward and a gift to others. Fighting the good fight for life can make us stronger, more resilient, teach us about ourselves, and help us discover things we might otherwise never have known.

Never giving up is what life is all about. If you would have given up the first time you crashed your bicycle, you would have never tried again. How about the first time you asked your spouse out and he or she said no; giving up would have not created a good, long, loving relationship, marriage and kids (if you have kids—we've got cats!)

Giving up isn't a part of our DNA. We are designed to grow, learn, experiment, fail, fall, and pick ourselves up again. We are designed to win, to keep going, inventing, creating, growing, and living life to our fullest potential. Never give up. Keep fighting for the right to live your life.

The cancer doesn't make you, create you, or control you. The cancer is a disease, a bad disease, and can be a deadly disease, but it's not you. Keep your eye on your dreams, your exciting future picture, the "should be" state not the "as is state."

Don't move into the cancer—move through it, stay your course, your purpose to live and enjoy life. The quote below can bring this thought process together. Don't stay with the cancer, move with it and through it if you're able. Don't live in it daily. Don't let the fears stop you from fighting and living. Don't allow fear to overcome your life.

What I feared most came to pass.
—The Book of Job

Change Is Okay

The next big "C" is all about change. Change is okay. It's what life is—daily change. There will always be change: change in the weather, change in our age, our hair color, and the seasons of life. Winter will always come and it will always follow fall, and spring will arrive, and then summer. Earth's cycles will continue to change. Our seasons of life will come and go—the seasons of earning, learning, and returning. In chess terms, it's the beginning game, the mid-game and the end game.

If you search, you will find that change is okay. Yes, the cancer journey will change you. It certainly changed me. Not all the change was for the bad; it was actually more good than bad, because I chose to look for the good, and turn the bad into good. I've found that if and when I search for the good, I can find it. (I've also learned that if I choose to search for the bad, that's just what I'll find.) It all depends on your attitude!

Change really is great. We see our children change and grow, our parents change, our friends or employees grow, and ourselves change. Change in this context is about accepting cancer and doing something good with it.

We live in changing times. Change is how we grow and develop ourselves to be better people. We can change our priorities, change our goals, and change our dreams. I've changed my goals from having a hot, fancy, fast car and earning a bazillion bucks to a much different way of thinking and purpose: it's now my season of returning and giving to others.

Don't let change scare you. Go for it, search it out, and make change exciting. We really never change until we change something that we do daily. Through change, we can change our world, which could change another person's world for the good. (How about that for a great book title? *Change is good… You go first!*)

Change is my passion, my quest, my daily habit, my drive. Change has taken me from the depths of living on the streets, from drug addiction, from being a high school dropout to becoming a good, giving person making a good living. Change has driven my success. Change has led me to Debbie. Change has been my motto, my life's journey. Change is what I've found living is all about. Change has helped me fight my cancer battle. If I could redo my life, "change" would be my middle name! I'm ready for daily change. What about you?

Change your thinking and you can change your life.

Encourage Others And Yourself

Learn to live life thoughtfully. Be gentle and thoughtful with others. Encourage them and enjoy the gift of life through others. By living life thoughtfully, you put the best interest of others first. One of my favorite adages is: You can get everything in life you want "IF" you help enough other people get what they want first.

I hope that you learn to live your life thoughtfully, thankfully, and faithfully.

The "E" means encourage others and encourage yourself. As a motivational speaker and professional development trainer, my life is all about encouragement. I've found that the more people I can encourage and offer hope, the better I feel. The better I feel about myself, the better my life will be.

The more we can be a blessing to others, the more blessings come our way. Cancer can throw a screw into the wheel of life. It can slow things down, and it can change your direction, thinking and mission. But cancer can also be encouraging, hopeful, possible, enlightening, and offer a new perspective on life. Self-encouragement is like motivation: the more we can encourage ourselves to fight the cancer, beat the chemotherapy, work through the radiation treatments, the better we can live life.

How do we live a better life? Answer: We work more on making ourselves better!

The ability to offer your story can be encouragement and motivation for others. Your drive and passion for life, can lift others and you to a higher level of enjoying life.

It's Not About Cancer; It's About You

Your cancer journey could be your new purpose in life—to lift another, offer hope to a person with a worse case of cancer or other illness. Your cancer may be your purpose-driven life, your reason for living, your mission to share your story of hope.

In climbing my mountain, I found that the little steps can make the big differences. Getting to the hospital every morning and making that four-hour round trip, taking the steps from the parking deck rather than the elevator, were my daily victories. I figured each step made me stronger and helped me with my physical recovery. Each step proved to me that I could keep moving, walking, and climbing my mountain.

What do you want to do with your cancer? You can't get rid of it, can't drop it off around the corner. There's no magic wand, no quick-fix program. Your cancer fight and daily victories can make the difference, even if it's just one victory a day, one treatment behind you. It's okay to take a bad thing and turn it into a good thing. Take your story to another person with cancer and share how you hit the wall, how big your wall was, and how you climbed the wall. Share how you looked at the mountain and decided to climb it and look back at your achievements. Share your victories, no matter how little or how big.

How can we take something as awful, as life-threatening, as cancer and see it as a gift of encouragement? Can one person's cancer journey offer hope to another? The answer is a resounding "Yes!"

We can make a difference in this big world. The world is much bigger than we are, but the cancer doesn't have to be bigger than us. Your ability to transfer the bad disease into a good tool of encouragement and hope is bigger than you think and bigger than the cancer. Make it happen!

Decide today to encourage others with or without cancer. Be a person of encouragement, a person who cares, a person of hope. There is something greater than cancer—YOU!

Reflect And Grow

Be happy with what you've got and where you are on your journey. Reflect and grow. That is my hope for you, to be happy with what you've got. Wherever you are, you now have something to give, some place to go to make a difference.

Reflect on your journey. Move out of the past and move out of regret. No camping out, no setting up house; just go visit when you need your own encouragement. When you need to remember where you've been and what you've accomplished, reflection is the method.

I was watching one of my (our) most favorite TV shows; *Criminal Minds* and heard this statement from David Rossi: "*Scars remind us of where we've been. They don't have to dictate where we're going or who we are."* Made me think of "Never give up", "Attitude is everything." It's not about the cancer, it is about me, where I'm going and who I am.

My hope for you is that you will beat your cancer, that you will laugh again, dance again, walk again, feel again, and enjoy your cancer-free life. I believe by being happy with what you've got is much more important than worrying about what you don't have.

You've got cancer or someone in your life has cancer. What's more important is who you've got in your corner. Love is bigger than cancer; love is stronger than the chemo, the radiation, and the medication. Your love for life is bigger than the cancer. Your dreams for your exciting future are your internal strength, your love for your children, spouse, parents, friends, your career, your life, are bigger than any cancer can get.

Reflection is good—it helps you realize how far you've come. Growth, hope, and purpose are what will help you climb your mountain and help others along their own personal climb.

As I come to the end of my message of encouragement and hope, I reflect back to the first day I noticed the lump, to the first meeting with my recovery team, to the day I got fitted for my radiation mask. I reflect back to my first day of chemotherapy and the fear I felt. I think about that hour lying on the cot in the surgery waiting room. I even reflect back on the disgusting piece of meatloaf a nurse pushed in front of me not even an hour after I came to—that had to be the worst part of my cancer surgery day!

I reflect back on the days of the feeding tube and the fear of even using it. I reflect back on the daily drive to and from my treatments. I just kept moving forward. I think back to the second night of my chemotherapy; it was a hard night, a scary night.

I look back to the fear I saw in Debbie's eyes that day in the meeting room with all those doctors, chemotherapy teams, radiation group, the surgeon. That day was one of the most stressful and scary days of my life—so many decisions that had to be made, and made fairly quickly. The love of my life was so scared, I knew then I needed to be the rock, the hope, and the encourager for both of us. It wasn't about me or the cancer—it was about Debbie.

When we make our dreams and hope bigger than cancer and when we make things about others, it gives us a magical, internal power to live and enjoy our gift of life. A life lived for others with purpose, even on our darkest and scariest days, is what life is all about, for me anyway.

As this book goes to print in the summer of 2011, over two years after my radiation and chemo treatments, I feel good. I've gained weight and I'm doing my best to live my life to my fullest potential, not only for me but more importantly, for Debbie and everyone who reads this little book of encouragement and hope.

I'll share with anyone I can encourage. I'm living my life; I'm not living the cancer life. I'm not living with the thoughts of "what if it comes back," I'm conquering my dreams, with a good attitude, never giving up, accepting that change will always occur and it's okay.

I'm living my life today encouraging others to the best of my ability. I'm making it my life's mission. I'm living my life by being happy with what I've got, and with what God has gifted me. I'm doing my very best to reflect and grow daily so that I can have much more to give along my life journey.

I'm now a "Cancer-Fighting Specialist," not just a professional speaker or a training specialist, but a lean, mean, cancer-fighting specialist, fighting for you and me, fighting for life and a purpose-driven life.

Please share your story with me at www.cancerfightingspecialist.com. I would love to hear about your mountain, your changes, and what these words have offered to you. We will all be together someday, cancer-free, fully enjoying our eternal lives. I can't wait to meet you, hug you, and talk with you. We can connect anytime—right now!

P.S. I wish you a wonderful life journey, full of many rewarding and awesome victories. Fight your good fight of faith and beat your cancer if you can, share your love, and enjoy your gift of life. Remember:

it's not about cancer it's about you

Sincerely,

Larry S. Cockerel

The Cancer-Fighting Specialist™ and
Expert on Aggressively Living Life™

acknowledgements

I wish to acknowledge those who have helped me with this book, my journey, and my life; it's not about cancer, it's about you, my Inner Circle. I thank everyone for your input, creativity, expertise, direction, and brutal honesty when I needed it. I read once that if you find a turtle on a fence post, you've got to know it didn't get there all by itself. Someone or something helped it get there. It's been the same with me; others helped me get here.

DEBBIE TACKES COCKEREL, my life partner, best friend, and leader of my "Cancer-Fighting Team" (including PeeWee,

Peanut, Whitey & Rocky; Whitey and Rocky both left us in 2009. Tough year!) As I write in 2011, this will be our 19th year together. I wouldn't change a thing about any of those years, even if I could. Debbie has always supported me with all my wild ideas and projects. I can't even imagine what my life would be like without her in mine.

With this book project, she helped me with research and cleaning up the screwed-up grammar and everything else on the pages that didn't look or sound right (and let me tell you, there was a lot!)

KIRA HENSCHEL, my publisher, for helping me to bring this book to the market. I thank Kira for her editorial skills, expertise, and guidance in pulling it all together. Kira has helped other speakers and trainers I know develop their books and I'm sure in the years to come, she will support many others in putting their stories in the hands of readers just like you. *www.HenschelHAUSBooks.com*

ANDREW WELYCZKO, the creative one behind the book. Andrew helped me develop the cover and came up with the interior design so my book flows visually. In the early days of coming up with the cover, Andrew had his thinking cap on and the emails flowed at the same rate as the creativity. Andrew was able to take my thoughts over email and phone and watching him put those on paper was exciting and awesome. Andrew has worked with other speakers I know and each final product looks great and inviting. *andrew@abandonedwest.com*

JASON LIENKE, with QuadGraphics, a great local printing and graphic company I've worked with for years. I can trust that Jason and his team will take my thoughts and ideas and develop them into something I can take to the market, whether it's my business cards, sell-sheets, or my tip booklets. I always appreciate the team's creativity and quick response time, even under pressure when I'm given short windows to develop a handout for a client. It's all about trust!
www.qg.com

DR. GREGORY HARTIG, M.D., FACS Professor, my surgeon at the University of Wisconsin–Madison Hospitals and Clinics. Dr. Hartig was referred to me over a lunch meeting and was key in beginning my journey as a cancer survivor. Dr. Hartig and his team helped me feel comfortable with the brutal facts, have trust with the process, and get ready to fight my battle. I would highly recommend this team to anyone.

DR. PAUL M. HARARI, M.D. Dr. Harari was head of my oncology team for the radiation treatments, and also worked with **DR. TIEN HOANG, M.D.,** Assistant Professor, and my chemotherapy doctor. Dr. Harari met with me weekly during my radiation treatments and kept a close eye on my progress and the process. The team at UW–Madison did everything to help me feel comfortable with all the changes going on in my life.

FACEBOOK FRIENDS. Just a short thank you to all my Facebook friends who encouraged me along my journey and helped me with ideas on cover design and provided me with lots of insights.

JOANNE BAKER (MY MOTHER). I give special thanks to my mother, who always believed in me, even in those years when there wasn't much to believe in. I know the love between a son and his mother cannot be put into words. Nor can the trust, the caring, the insight, and the faith my mother has had in me. My mother was there with me the night before and the day of my surgery, along with her husband, Gerald Baker, my brother David De Block, my sister Rene Stephens, and my niece Kristen Stephens. With Debbie there, my "Cancer-Fighting Team" was created!

I love you, Mother. You have always been my strength, my rock.

ROBERT IAN. Robert is a colleague from the National Speakers Association–Wisconsin, Past President of our Chapter and the one who met with me over lunch at Taco John's in Madison, WI to talk about NSA and my succession to President. Then right before my eyes, the conversation led to my connection with UW–Madison, my surgeon and the medical team who helped me get to where I am today. Who says that there isn't a God, a power greater than you and I? That day was just not another day, not just a coincidence; more like a miracle and a taco! I suggest you check Robert out at his website, get his book, and hire him for one of your future conferences.

www.conquerchange.com

about the author

Larry S. Cockerel, a.k.a. The Cancer-Fighting Specialist™ and The Sales Development Pro™, invests his time as a training specialist for business leaders and sales professionals by helping them maximize their results. As a professional speaker, Larry motivates and inspires people to maximize their potential, master change, and live life to their fullest potential.

Larry lives in Cedarburg, Wisconsin with Debbie and their two "kids" (cats), enjoying life to their fullest potential.

When not training and speaking, Larry spends his time reading and writing, enjoys listening to music, riding with

Debbie on their Harley, and eating out! As a cancer survivor, Larry's mission is to offer hope and encouragement to everyone he meets!

He is available to speak or offer workshops for your organization or event. Just visit Larry at www.larrycockerel.com and www.cancerfightingspecialist.com.

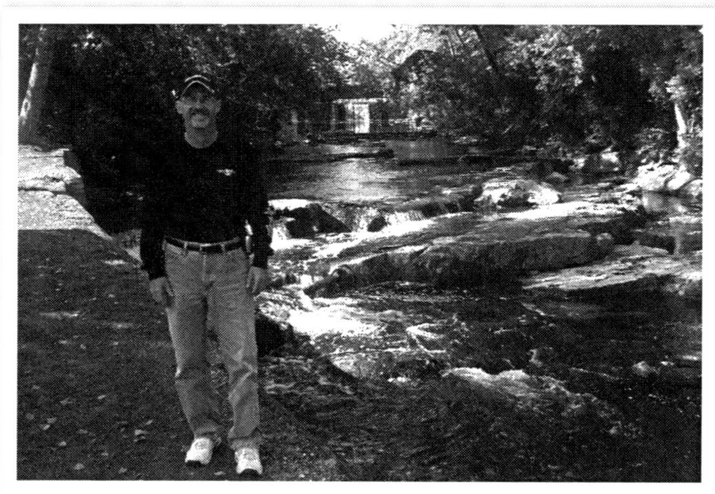

Please share your story with Larry at:

WWW.CANCERFIGHTINGSPECIALIST.COM

He truly would like to hear from you.

appendix

squamous cell carcinoma

In the United States, squamous cell carcinoma of the head and neck comprises about 4 percent of all malignancies. This corresponds to an estimated 17 per 100,000 persons with newly diagnosed squamous cell carcinoma of the head and neck per year. Male-to-female incidence rates are greater than 3:1. The discrepancy in the male-to-female ratio is even more pronounced in laryngeal tumors, in which carcinoma is 4 to 5 times more common in men. This ratio has declined in the last 20 years, possibly reflecting the increased number of women using tobacco products during this period.

Information courtesy of the American Cancer Society.

Squamous cell carcinoma represents more than 90 percent of all head and neck cancers. A malignant tumor of epithelial origin, squamous cell carcinoma has a regional distribution involved in the biological activity of the neoplasm. Behavior of squamous cell cancer depends on its site of origin

History

Evidence of head and neck carcinomas has been found in ancient skulls. The oldest known tumor is contained in a fossil found in east Africa by Richard Leakey that dates back more than 500,000 years. Some historians speculate that a high incidence of nasopharyngeal cancer may have been present in some ancient populations because of the inhalation of wood smoke in poorly ventilated huts. In approximately 400 BC, Hippocrates described a common chronic ulcer at the edge of the tongue that he attributed to the presence of sharp teeth rubbing against the tongue.

The ancient Indian physician Sushruta described the removal of tumors and developed great skill in plastic surgery, partly from defects created by frequent amputations of the nose and ears for punishment. Modern Western medicine received its foundation from early Roman medical writings. Little medical advancement was made for head and neck cancers until the advent of anesthesia and surgical excision in the 11th century.

In 1893, President Grover Cleveland was found to have a squamous cell carcinoma of the hard palate that required surgical excision. The operation was performed secretly on a yacht so that he could manage the "financial panic of 1893." Cleveland was known for his heavy cigar smoking and social drinking.

Cancer Remission

This is a topic that I didn't discuss in my book, and I'm not sure why, being that the phrase is tied so closely to cancer. Excuse me if you will, please. I guess the reason I didn't sprinkle this phrase throughout the book is that I don't want to believe in the meaning as I understand it. I don't want to live my life thinking, "Well, it's coming back. I'm just in my remission." To me that isn't positive thinking with the right attitude.

The politically correct meaning from the American Cancer Society (ACS) is: "a period of time when the cancer is responding to treatment or is under control. In a complete cancer remission, all the signs and symptoms of the disease disappear... Complete cancer remissions may continue for several years and be considered cures." So, someone who goes into cancer remission is not showing signs or symptoms of the cancer. It doesn't matter how many cancer cells are still going strong and growing in the body of the patient. For any time frame that it isn't causing "signs and symptoms," the patient is said to be in remission.

I hope that any of my readers who have been touched by cancer is either in remission or totally free of this terrible and frightening disease. God bless all my readers. Live your life conquering your dreams and enjoying your gift of life!

Hear my cry, O God; attend to my prayer.

From the end of the earth I will cry to You,
when my heart is overwhelmed;
lead me to the rock that is higher than I.

For You have been a shelter for me,
a strong tower from the enemy.
I will abide in Your tabernacle forever;
I will trust in the shelter of Your wings.

◆　◆　◆

Psalms 61: 1–4